Yoga Therapy for Stroke

Yoga Therapy
for Stroke

A Handbook for Yoga Therapists
and Healthcare Professionals

ARLENE A. SCHMID and
MARIEKE VAN PUYMBROECK

Forewords by Matthew J. Taylor and Linda S. Williams

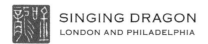

SINGING DRAGON
LONDON AND PHILADELPHIA

First published in 2019
by Singing Dragon
an imprint of Jessica Kingsley Publishers
73 Collier Street
London N1 9BE, UK
and
400 Market Street, Suite 400
Philadelphia, PA 19106, USA

www.singingdragon.com

Library of Congress Cataloging in Publication Data
A CIP catalog record for this book is available from the Library of Congress

British Library Cataloguing in Publication Data
A CIP catalogue record for this book is available from the British Library

ISBN 978 1 84819 369 7
eISBN 978 0 85701 327 9

Printed and bound in Great Britain

The handouts marked with ☑ can be downloaded to print
from www.jkp.com/voucher using the code XEOKYDY.

Contents

Foreword

Stroke. Both a noun and a verb. The old English is a "gentle caress." The clinical diagnosis? A swift, silent swipe through a human life that affects every part of that life and the entire community fabric of which they are an interconnected thread. *Yoga Therapy for Stroke* masterfully unfolds this paradoxical word for the reader to discover not only the lived experience of the person with the diagnosis, but also the opportunities and challenges for those of us that are related or hope to serve in their processing of healing.

It is no surprise to me that Doctors Schmid and Van Puymbroeck have proven themselves up to this task. Arlene and Marieke have been yoga/rehabilitation colleagues and friends of mine for years in an initially small, but growing cadre of like-minded professionals. While their academic pedigree carries the title "Doctor," one only need spend a few minutes with them and you sense their enormous hearts and spirits that make such formality feel stiff and awkward. Their book sheds that same quality of warmth and compassion as they balance their academic and clinical brilliance with a writing style that is accessible for their varied audience of yoga professionals, rehabilitation professionals, and front-line support providers.

The power of a stroke demands this inclusive spirit of theirs. That swift, silent swipe through the neurological architecture of the individual is a transformative wound. The event is what the late Irish poet John O'Donohue described as a "threshold" in life. Suddenly, everything changes as the person steps across the threshold from the room of "before stroke" into the new room of "after stroke." Quite literally their wound changes their brain's form (trans-forms). So too does every relationship they have: self, family, occupation, social roles, avocations, spiritual, and on and on. Each of the relationships is forever altered and without care can be separated if not reconnected or "yoked" back together. What better reason do we need to dive in and explore how yoga (the science of yoking/connecting) can serve to transform a wound of the marvelous brain from "broken" to what O'Donohue describes as a "sacred wound"?

Please don't be alarmed those of you of a more conservative or conventional perspective. "Sacred" doesn't mean something religious, and what this book teaches is neither woo-woo nor a threat to anyone's spiritual practice. Rather, sacred means "to make holy/whole," the opposite of profane or common. In our conventional rehabilitation world, injury and illness is approached as something to get over, past, or beyond.

A stroke doesn't afford us that privilege. Even if a full recovery of function is achieved, nothing in that person's life is ever the same again. That's what transformative means. Yoga differs in approach to injury and illness. It does not treat or cure. Yoga does not seek to get over, past, or beyond. A practice that invites and explores both reflection and action based on that attention restores the new relationships affected, making the wound whole or sacred. To not attend to every aspect is both profane and incomplete.

As you will read, yoga is such a practice of attention and invites a pause to right now, this moment, this breath, for all of us to ask, "What is?" Not what was, and not what will be, just, "What is?" It is that simple, and that hard.

The authors have also successfully avoided teaching just "parts" of yoga in isolation, which would produce additional fragmentation of care. You are about to discover the full spectrum of what makes up yoga, not just some new exercises to add to therapy. It doesn't matter whether you are the person who had the stroke, the one providing support, or the one teaching the practices, the good news is you can't help but care for yourself as well when you employ *Yoga Therapy for Stroke*. As you read, then practice and experience, you will be slowing, sensing and waking up to "What is?" right now, creating space for your own health, but also priming for the creativity that stroke demands from each of us.

Arlene and Marieke have set us up to claim the healing creativity that exists in each of us. They are collectively redefining their professions as well by this work. Arlene, as an "occupy-ational" therapist, has stepped forward in her already comprehensive tradition to prod her colleagues to offer even deeper exploration of how their patients and themselves as therapists "occupy" this moment by advocating the inclusion of yoga therapeutically in personal and professional practice. Marieke invites her peers as "re-creational" therapists to step forward and assume their full agency to create environments where their patients "re-create" their lives in this new, post-stroke room of life. And both aren't just being wishful but continue to "walk the talk" through the rigorous asana of research, making their vision real in a way that will transform the conventional healthcare body of literature.

For the yoga professionals reading, you have a special treat ahead. The design of this book ensures a very practical understanding of how your yoga can safely weave into supporting students and their caregivers. The yoga practice of ahimsa (non-violence) is reinforced through the book so that you and your clientele can be safe. No matter if you are sitting with your first student post-stroke, or have taught for years as an early pioneer, there is much to discover in the pages ahead.

In closing, may I encourage each of us to model what the authors do every day: reach out to your local community to learn from one another, forge respectful interprofessional communication, and remember the people that have had a stroke are both the experts and our teachers.

Together, may we all work towards Patanjali's Yoga Sutra 2.16:

Heyam duhkham anagatam: Prevent the suffering that is yet to come.

Yoga Therapy for Stroke brings us that much closer.

Matthew J. Taylor, PT, PhD, C-IAYT
Founder and Director of SmartSafeYoga

Foreword

Stroke is common, familiar to healthcare practitioners and lay persons alike, and yet also strikingly individual, as it affects each person in a unique way. Because each person is a unique amalgamation of their physical, mental, emotional, social, and spiritual selves, and because each stroke is unique in location and size, the effects of stroke on the whole person are complex and changing over time.

At its core, stroke represents a sudden fracturing of the mind-body connection, often causing unexpected physical difficulties as what was physically subconscious becomes consciously effortful. Equally if not more difficult is the frequent effect on self-image, as stroke survivors experience a loss of knowing the self and knowing one's place in the world. Decades of brain research have clearly shown that physical and cognitive therapies are effective in harnessing the brain's natural systems of plasticity after stroke, promoting network repair and formation and improving stroke survivors' function and well-being. Yoga, as a practice that harnesses both mind and body, is ideally positioned to mend this fracture.

Drs. Schmid and Van Puymbroeck have, in *Yoga Therapy for Stroke*, generously shared their wealth of experience as therapists, clinical researchers, and yoga practitioners and teachers so that the seemingly daunting possibility of bringing yoga to the stroke survivor is made possible. They give proven, practical advice and example practices for therapists who want to integrate yoga into their therapeutic practice, for yogis who want to integrate differently abled stroke survivors into their yoga classes, and for stroke survivors themselves who are looking for ways to guide themselves into greater recovery. This book is critically important for all of these audiences, as therapists and yogis need additional tools to offer, and stroke survivors need access to evidence-based therapeutic interventions beyond those typically offered in a medical setting.

Integrating yoga into post-stroke care and recovery is a practice desperately in need of implementation across healthcare systems and communities. Having experienced firsthand the impact this practice has had on my own stroke patients, I am thrilled that Arlene and Marieke's expertise will now reach a wider audience. *Yoga Therapy for Stroke* offers a way for all of us to take this next step, which will undoubtedly lead to sustainable improvements in the care and recovery for stroke survivors. For physicians like me, this book will expand the horizons of what you recommend for your patients, hopefully leading you to work within your system of practice to promote the adoption of yoga for stroke survivors. For yoga instructors, this book will encourage you to increasingly offer your wisdom to stroke survivors and those with other physical challenges. For stroke survivors and their loved ones, this book will empower you to approach recovery in a way that supports your whole self…mind, body, and spirit. For all of us, and especially for the stroke survivor, this book embodies the words of B. K. Iyengar, internationally known yogi and practitioner of adapted yoga after his own spinal injury: "Yoga teaches us to cure what need not be endured and endure what cannot be cured." Namaste.

Linda S. Williams
Professor of Neurology, Indiana University School of Medicine

Acknowledgments

Arlene: We are so thankful to Betty Svendsen for being part of this book and our yoga lives. Betty was a participant in a study here in Fort Collins, CO, and was our model for many of the photos. She had a stroke and was excited to use yoga as part of her recovery. In addition, we thank Aaron Eakman, PhD, OTR for being our photographer for the photos included of Betty. Aaron is also an occupational therapist and faculty at Colorado State University. His son Garrett was also so helpful and patient with our photo shoot! Finally, we thank Meraki Yoga (https://merakiyogastudio.com) for donating the space for the photo shoot, and for their excitement regarding the development of accessible yoga programming in our community. And I am so grateful for my husband, BZ, and all of your support during this and all the phases of my life! We are SO lucky… xoxo

Marieke: We are also so grateful for the outstanding models, Charity Hubbard and Abby Wiles. They are both MS students in the Clemson University Recreational Therapy Program and very active members of the Yoga Research Team. They are a joy to work with! The amazing Em Adams, MS, CTRS, C-IAYT came to the Clemson campus to work on her PhD at the perfect time to help us, along with her husband Brian, to capture the pictures for the chapters about asanas, restorative yoga, and mudra. Em's vast knowledge as a C-IAYT helped tremendously in the writing of Chapter 6 on the description and modifications of asanas for yoga post-stroke, as well as other chapters. Em, thanks so much for all that you did to make this project a success! We are so grateful! Also, thank you so much to Julie Vidotto, who let us use the beautiful OLLI facility for our photo shoot! And to my sweet Charles: every day with you is a blessing. Thanks for your unwavering love and support. xoxo

We are so grateful that we met each other in 2001 at the University of Florida. We quickly hit it off and have been working and playing together ever since. [Arlene: You are the best friend a girl could ask for—this is such a fun and exciting adventure to be on with you!] [Marieke: We have learned so much from each other and from this experience! We are so lucky to be doing this together! Xoxo!]

We are so grateful to Dr. Matthew Taylor and Dr. Linda Williams for believing in us and taking time to write poignant forewords for this book. We really appreciate your support.

CHAPTER 1

Introduction

"The glory of friendship is not the outstretched hand, not the kindly smile, nor the joy of companionship; it is the spiritual inspiration that comes to one when you discover that someone else believes in you and is willing to trust you with a friendship."

Ralph Waldo Emerson

Mission of the Book

The mission of this book is to teach healthcare professionals, including rehabilitation and yoga therapists, the art of using yoga as an approach to rehabilitation, recovery, and healing after stroke.

Why Us?

Arlene A. Schmid, PhD, OTR, FAOTA, RYT-200

I grew up in Buffalo, NY, in the United States, and early on knew I wanted to be an occupational therapist. When I completed my college education to be an occupational therapist, I also knew I wanted to see new things and live somewhere warmer. I moved to Honolulu, Hawaii, where I began working as an occupational therapist in a variety of settings. I quickly learned that there was a large influence of Eastern medicine and philosophies in healthcare and day-to-day life in Hawaii; this included yoga being everywhere. Yoga and Eastern medicine was a completely new way for me to view and understand my surroundings, and I dove in to yoga head first! I personally began to learn yoga and immediately fell in love with it; it was good for my heart and soul and for my physical body. I then began to learn about teaching yoga and some basic yogic philosophies and then, without really thinking about it, I began to use yoga in my clinical occupational therapy practice. I worked in a variety of settings as an occupational therapist, including working in skilled nursing facilities, adolescent mental health, and hand therapy. When I began to use yoga with many different clients, I found it interesting that yoga often helped different people for different reasons. I knew yoga was working, but I didn't know why, and I knew there was a need, and an opportunity, to research the benefits of yoga for people with different disabilities.

After living in Hawaii, and really loving it, I decided I wanted to further explore the use of yoga, and the benefits of yoga, for people with disabilities. I made the difficult decision to leave Hawaii and move to Florida to attend the University of Florida. There I earned my PhD in Rehabilitation Science and began working on rehabilitation intervention research related to people with stroke. Over the decade following the completion of my PhD, I spent many years learning about people with stroke and their needs. I studied the development of fear of falling in people with stroke and learned that fall prevention was an important, but unaddressed, issue for people with stroke. With my colleague, Marieke, I began to run research studies about the benefits of yoga for older adults, women with breast cancer, and then finally with stroke. We have now run many yoga studies, for people with many kinds of disabilities, and we have learned so much! Our research tells us that yoga leads to many improvements for many people, and especially for people with stroke. We have learned that people with chronic stroke, people who had a stroke over 25 years ago, can still change and can still improve! Importantly, we have also learned that it is feasible to include yoga for clients during their rehabilitation, and that people, even with the most severe disabilities, can still complete and benefit from yoga.

In this book, we hope to offer yoga and rehabilitation therapists and other health professionals ways to safely use yoga and integrate yoga into clinical practice. We are addressing all kinds of therapists, including, but not limited to, occupational therapists, recreational therapists, physical therapists, and, importantly, yoga therapists. We hope that we offer a holistic intervention that treats the mind and the body and that allows for physical, cognitive, and emotional improvements, but also improves the clients' abilities to accept their new bodies and live in the moment, allowing them to recover to their fullest abilities.

I now live happily in Fort Collins, CO, surrounded by mountains and yoga. I spend my time with my husband (BZ) and two dogs, playing and working hard. We love to hike, bike, kayak, and, of course, do some yoga. I recently completed my 200-hour yoga teacher training, and the focus of the training was Viniyoga. Viniyoga is considered to be a therapeutic style of Hatha yoga. I chose Viniyoga as it is therapeutic and is based on normal development patterns of movement. Viniyoga is a Sanskrit word that implies adaptation or appropriate application, perfect for an occupational therapist! I am so grateful that I completed my yoga teacher training, I learned so much about myself and am sure that it has positively impacted my yoga research and my day-to-day life.

For clinicians who are using yoga as part of their clinical practice, I highly encourage becoming involved with the International Association of Yoga Therapists (www.iayt.org). This is not limited to yoga therapists but is for all therapists (i.e. occupational therapists, recreational therapists, physical therapists) who are using yoga. The organization hosts two meetings a year, one focused on education and one focused on academic research.

Marieke Van Puymbroeck, PhD, CTRS, FDRT, LVCYT, RYT-500

I found yoga during my first academic job at the University of Illinois. I had just graduated from the University of Florida with a PhD in Rehabilitation Science and was looking for inspiration for my new academic research line, as well as new recreation for myself. My research had been focused on caregivers of individuals with stroke, and I had done a lot of big secondary data analysis, but I was ready to do what recreational therapists do—work with people using recreation as an intervention! I was not sure how to make the transition to intervention research, but my mind was open to any possibility. Yoga was not on my radar at all, but I met a great yoga teacher, Jenna Cameron Juday, at a garage sale who told me about the Vinyasa yoga class she offered nearby. During Downward Facing Dog in my very first yoga class, I realized the power that yoga has to make people feel so much better! I felt great, and I had a hunch that it would make caregivers feel great also! From that first hunch, I was funded to start a research program using yoga as a therapeutic intervention for informal caregivers. Shortly thereafter, Arlene moved to the Midwest, and we began to marry our research efforts using yoga as a therapeutic intervention for women with breast cancer, older adults with a fear of falling, individuals with stroke, and, in the past ten years, we have studied the use of yoga with many other neurological populations.

As a recreational therapist and rehabilitation scientist, I am a firm believer in the power that recreation activities, such as yoga, have to improve the overall functioning of an individual. Our research and others' have borne out that yoga, an ancient practice, has many modern-day implications for health and well-being. By combining physical postures (asanas), breath work (pranayama), meditation (dhyana), and hand positions (mudras), the body and mind respond by joining together to improve the health of the practitioner.

My first yoga teacher training was in Lakshmi Voelker chair yoga. Lakshmi is an amazing force and spirit, and she and her husband have dedicated their lives to making yoga accessible for everyone. Chair yoga can be a vigorous practice and can yield similar benefits to a standing practice, but it removes a lot of perceived obstacles by having people sit during the entire practice. With that certification under my belt, I completed my 200-hour teacher training at Asheville Yoga Center in Asheville, NC. During my nine-month program, I was so fortunate to be surrounded by an amazing cohort of lovely folks, including four other rehabilitation therapists. During the process, I learned even more about myself than I did about yoga. That being said, learning the details of the philosophy, the history, and specific yogic strategies was superbly helpful and influential in understanding the magic that is yoga. I was also introduced to Kundalini yoga during this teacher training and have since spent a number of weeks dedicated to learning more and immersing in this ancient practice. I have completed my 300-hour advanced teacher training at Asheville Yoga Center. I am so grateful for the spectacular teachers I have had the honor of learning from, including Sierra Hollister, Michael Johnson, and Libby Hinsey (all from Asheville Yoga Center). Doug Keller's deep knowledge of the therapeutic wisdom of yoga has really been pivotal in my life. I have also learned a lot from Seane Corne—her social justice and activism via yoga speak to my heart. Dianne Bondy is an inspiration to me—she is an all-round rad individual who I had the opportunity to meet at the Accessible Yoga Conference. If you are interested in making yoga accessible to all people, check out the Accessible Yoga Conference. I also had the great opportunity to spend a lot of time with Peggy Ambler, a yoga therapist (C-IAYT) and physical therapy assistant, who trained me in advanced restorative yoga and the use of hot stones in restorative yoga. She spent a lot of time working with me, and I am grateful.

A Note from Both of Us

In today's world, many people think that yoga is only for lithe, young women. Importantly, this is not the case. Yoga can improve the health of anyone and can be modified to meet people where they are, regardless of health conditions or limitations. In this book, we rely on our rehabilitation experience and knowledge, as well as our well-tested experience in working with people with stroke, to provide modifications that are appropriate for people with varying levels of ability, as well as options for the therapist to assist and instruct mental practice if the physicality of the postures is not available. We are excited to share with you the benefit of yoga for people with stroke.

See Figure 1.1 of us doing yoga together in Rocky Mountain State Park in Colorado!

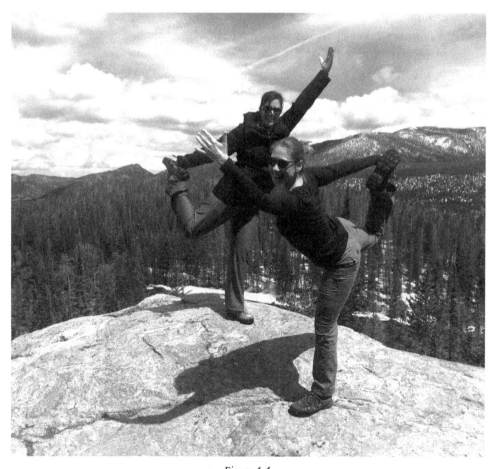

Figure 1.1

We attempted to write Chapters 2 and 3 with multiple professionals in mind: the yoga therapist or the yoga teacher who may have limited experience working with clients with stroke but a vast knowledge of yoga; and healthcare professionals, such as rehabilitation therapists, who may have extensive experience in working with clients with stroke, but less experience in adding yoga to their clinical practice. Therefore, we provide information about stroke and stroke-related disability in Chapter 2 and about yoga, including yogic philosophies, in Chapter 3.

We invite you on the journey to include yoga in your practice with individuals who have had a stroke. There are so many potential benefits for this population, and we hope that this book will be a useful guide for you. Namaste.

The handouts featured in Chapters 12 and 13 can be downloaded to print from www.jkp.com/voucher using the code XEOKYDY.

CHAPTER 2

Exploring Stroke Basics

A REVIEW AND PRIMER

Most rehabilitation therapists, such as occupational, physical, and recreational therapists, will have a relatively firm understanding of stroke and the consequences of stroke. Therefore, this chapter will likely be a review of stroke content for the rehabilitation therapists. In contrast, the yoga teacher or the yoga therapist may have less knowledge about stroke; therefore, in this chapter, we provide a review of stroke statistics and stroke-related disability, and touch on the use of yoga for clients with stroke. Yoga, and its use after stroke, is greatly expounded upon in future chapters.

Stroke is a complex medical event that greatly disrupts the life of your client who has sustained a stroke, as well as the lives of their family and friends. After a stroke, it may sometimes look like only the physical body is impacted, but it is essential for you, the yoga or rehabilitation therapist, to understand that stroke also may lead to cognitive and emotional disabilities, many of which may be addressed through yoga. In this chapter, we will discuss: the disconnect between the mind and the body that seems to be a common occurrence after a stroke; pertinent information related to stroke; and the residual disability that may occur after a stroke. As appropriate, we also include information about yoga as therapy after a stroke or how the therapist may best manage different aspects of post-stroke disability.

What Is a Stroke?

A stroke is often called a "brain attack," because it is similar to a heart attack but occurs in the brain. A stroke damages the blood vessels, known as arteries, that take blood away from the heart and to the brain (among other areas of the body). Arteries bring blood to the brain; the blood, coming from the heart, includes oxygen and nutrients that the brain needs to function. A stroke occurs because the artery is blocked or ruptures and, subsequently, the brain does not receive the blood, oxygen, and nutrients that it needs. When this happens, brain cells die, and a part of the brain dies. Disability that occurs after a stroke is different, dependent on the size and location of the damage to the specific area of the brain. It is important to also understand that stroke is not a progressive or deteriorating disease like multiple sclerosis or Parkinson's Disease.

After a stroke, people typically plateau in their recovery after approximately one year, but, due to neuroplasticity allowing for additional recovery, they can also still make improvements for many years post-stroke.

Neuroplasticity

Neuroplasticity is a reality for people with stroke. While we know that parts of the brain are damaged by a stroke, we also know that the brain and the pathways in the brain can heal and can change or reorganize. Neuroplasticity allows for these changes and means that a new pathway can form or adjust in the brain and that people with stroke can learn or relearn important movements and skills. While a lot of the natural recovery that happens after a stroke occurs in the first 6 to 12 months after the stroke, neuroplasticity allows for continued changes to happen long after the stroke. Thanks to neuroplasticity, we have certainly seen 90-year-old people or people with strokes from 20 years ago see great improvement after yoga.

Types of Stroke

In our yoga studies, we have included clients with different types of stroke (Schmid, *et al.*, 2012, 2014, 2016b). We have not seen differences in study outcomes related to type or location of stroke. In general, we see improvements across all clients, regardless of stroke type or location. Each client is of course different, but we have found that modified yoga postures, breath work, meditation, and mantras can be used in therapy with all clients with stroke.

There are two primary types of stroke, ischemic and hemorrhagic. *Ischemic strokes* are much more common, with up to 87% of all strokes being ischemic (American Stroke Association, 2017). An ischemic stroke is when there is a clot or a blockage in a blood vessel that supplies blood to a part of the brain. There are multiple blood vessels, or arteries, that supply the brain with blood. Each vessel supplies a different part of the brain, and the artery that is blocked will determine the part of the brain that has a stroke or the result of the stroke.

Hemorrhagic strokes occur when a blood vessel ruptures or bleeds into the brain. A blood vessel rupture typically occurs when a person has a blood vessel or artery that is weakened. Two kinds of hemorrhagic stroke exist: an intracerebral hemorrhagic stroke occurs within the brain and a subarachnoid hemorrhagic stroke happens when the bleed occurs between the brain and the tissue that covers or surrounds the brain. Brain bleeds add pressure to the brain, resulting in damage. Finally, a person may sustain a *transient ischemic attack*. This is generally considered a "mini" stroke and it is thought that the transient ischemic attack does not typically result in permanent damage to the brain. A transient ischemic attack is a primary risk factor for a future stroke.

Some Stroke Statistics

- Every two seconds, somewhere in the world, someone has a stroke.

- In the United Kingdom, nearly 100,000 people sustain a stroke annually, and nearly 800,000 people have a stroke annually in the United States.

- Stroke is the fourth leading cause of death in the United Kingdom and fifth leading cause of death in the United States.

- It is thought that up to 80% of strokes are preventable (see Chapter 14 for information about preventing future strokes, including how yoga supports the prevention of stroke through improvement of blood pressure, stress, and other stroke risk factors). Modifiable stroke risk factors include: diet, physical activity, blood pressure, and managing stress.

- Stroke is the leading cause of long-term disability in the United States and, in the United Kingdom, is one of the largest causes of disability.

- Approximately two thirds of people who sustain and survive a stroke are living with some residual impairment or disability.

- Stroke is the most commonly seen diagnosis by rehabilitation therapists.

(American Stroke Association, 2016; Stroke Association, 2018)

The Mind-Body Disconnect After Stroke

Often, there seems to be a disconnect between the mind and the body after a stroke (Garrett, Immink, and Hillier, 2011). Through our clinical practice and in our studies, we have worked with many people who have sustained a stroke, and we too notice the disconnect between the mind and the body. This change in the mind and body connection is likely secondary to the post-stroke cerebral damage (Garrett, Immink, and Hillier, 2011). The damage to the brain means that multiple body systems are compromised. The complex systems of the brain and body require integration of the mind and multiple body functions, structures, and systems to work most effectively (Weerdesteyn, *et al.*, 2008). We propose that an intervention that involves a holistic mind and body intervention and is capable of simultaneously targeting multiple systems, such as yoga, would be effective post-stroke. Yoga is one of the few interventions that targets multiple body systems that are compromised after stroke and provides an integrative set of practices consistent with treating the whole body.

In addition to the damage to the brain, a traumatic event (think about post-traumatic stress) may also lead to a mind-body disconnect. A stroke is certainly traumatic for the individual who sustained the stroke and for their family. However, we think that the mind-body disconnect after a stroke is also exacerbated by the subsequent disability that occurs as secondary to the stroke. For example, if someone has post-stroke hemiparesis and cannot feel or move a leg or arm as they previously could, it stands to reason that they may become disconnected from that limb or even angry at the limb. We see people who seem to forget to use their arm or their leg. We also have worked with many people who are very angry at their arm or their leg and are often angry because the limb does not work quite right or at all. We know that it feels as if the body is not listening, and we understand that it must be very frustrating for people.

Collectively, all of these changes in the brain and the body, the trauma of the stroke, and the new stroke-related disability seem to leave a disconnect between the mind and the body. We know that yoga and meditation can reconnect the mind and the body. This is likely related to the pairing of movement with the breath and focusing on the breath. Yoga means yolk—to unite. Yoga can help to merge the disconnect, to connect the mind and body after stroke. We know that not everyone can move through a yoga posture independently. But we also think, through our clinical practice and our research, that yoga can help with the disconnect through:

- mental practice of postures with breath (see Chapter 5)

- helping facilitate the movement through the posture and modifying yoga postures (see Chapter 6)

- connecting the breath with the movement.

There Is No "Bad Arm"

Perhaps related to the mind-body disconnect, for some reason, it is very common for people with stroke to refer to their affected extremity as the "bad" arm or the "bad" leg. This may come from the family talking like this or a healthcare provider or therapist using this language. We firmly believe that this language of calling part of the body "bad" is detrimental to the person with stroke and to their recovery and may lead to a further mind-body disconnect. Time and again we have worked with clients who use this language; they also express frustration or anger about their body part. We also hear this language from other therapists, friends, students, nurses, and doctors, and we wish to change this. It is common that after a stroke the body does not work the way it did prior to the stroke, and that the person needs to learn to live with a new body. Often there is motor and sensory impairment after stroke, meaning that people cannot move in the same way or feel things in the same way as before they had their stroke. However, we think that when the individual is so angry at their limb for not doing or feeling the right things, they begin to disconnect from their body. We think that people cannot recover to their fullest potential if they have this mind-body disconnect or if they are angry at their body. Likely adding to the disconnect, people may begin to ignore their limb or body part as it does not respond the way they want to. When the limb is not used, there is further loss of connectivity in the brain. Some people may have something called left neglect, when the mind ignores or neglects the left side of the body. Regardless of the reason, we highly encourage all therapists, healthcare providers, and family members to never use the word "bad" when referring to a limb or body part. Consider using the words "right" or "left" or saying "the affected arm." Give tactile cues to remind the client of their limb. Give them verbal cues if you are touching their right or left arm or leg. We think these cues help to reintegrate the mind and the body, thus beginning to address the mind-body disconnect that may happen after the stroke.

Differentiating Between the Left and Right Side of the Body

Many of the people with stroke who we have worked with seem to have some trouble knowing their left from their right. This too may be related to the mind-body disconnect that we witness. Not knowing the left side from the right side impacts how the yoga or rehabilitation therapist provides cueing in yoga during the physical postures. For people who have trouble knowing their left from their right, we find it helpful to use physical touch as a cue. We also might just say to "raise an arm" and allow the client to decide which limb to move, but we also make sure the client goes through the yoga postures with both sides of the body. Over time, we have seen improvements in people knowing their left from right and being able to follow directions related to each side of the body.

The "What If"

After working with many people with stroke, we have learned that people may get a bit stuck in the "what if." The brain being stuck in the "what if" may further widen the mind-body disconnect after a stroke. By the "what if" we mean that we have heard people say, "What if I exercised more?" or "What if I ate less fish and chips?" or "What if I listened to my doctor?" or "What if I didn't have a stroke?" We totally understand this and know that a stroke is a life-changing event. However, we also know that people tend to get stuck here, and we really believe that the rumination on the "what if" may hinder one's ability to fully move on to recovery. *Rumination* is overthinking or simply the repeat of thoughts over and over again. If someone is spending all of their time thinking about what happened or what they could have changed, it does not leave a lot of room for the future and for recovery. We also believe that yoga, including meditation or mantras, helps to control the rumination and allows for improved recovery and outcomes. We have seen people with stroke from over 20 years ago who are still devastated about the stroke and the losses they sustained. But after yoga and helping to change the mind-set, we see people becoming more accepting of their post-stroke body and lives. And it seems that once people are more accepting of who and where they are, they are able to also see some improvement in cognitive, emotional, and physical outcomes, or at least be more satisfied with who they are.

Stroke-Related Disability

Disability after a stroke is complex and looks different for different people. Often, we may think of stroke disability as being something we can see or a physical disability. We may see someone with a different walking or gait pattern, we may see someone have trouble using a spoon and getting food to their mouth, or we may see someone have trouble chewing and swallowing food. But, related to the type and location of the stroke and the severity of the stroke, there is often "hidden" disability, such as changes in cognitive abilities or emotions, including increased risk of depression. Some level of natural recovery of some of these specific stroke-related changes is common during the acute phases of stroke. Rehabilitation has traditionally been included after stroke to further facilitate recovery. Recently, researchers have shown that yoga may positively impact many post-stroke-related cognitive, emotional, and physical disabilities. We provide information regarding cognitive, emotional, and physical disabilities that the yoga or rehabilitation therapist is likely to see when working with clients with stroke, as well as possible tips for incorporating yoga when these issues do in fact manifest. For additional information on post-stroke-related disabilities, consider visiting these websites:

- Stroke Association: www.stroke.org.uk/what-stroke/common-problems-after-stroke

- American Heart Association: www.strokeassociation.org/STROKEORG/AboutStroke/About-Stroke_UCM_308529_SubHomePage.jsp.

Yoga may improve various aspects of stroke-related disability, including cognitive, emotional, and physical changes. Proven with medical scans of the brain, meditation has been shown to improve connectivity in the brain, as well as the actual size or thickness of the cortical matter (Lazar *et al.*, 2000, 2005). Because a stroke will damage a part of the brain, it is thought that yoga and meditation may be useful to heal or alter part of the damage. Yoga, as discussed throughout this book, includes meditation, physical postures, and breath work. In general, yoga may potentially lead to post-stroke improvements through: increasing or altering blood flow to the brain; enhancing cross-hemisphere blood flow (partly through crossing the midline of the body with eyes, arms, and legs); calming the nervous system; integrating new movement patterns; changing neural pathways; grounding the mind and body; and reconnecting the mind and body.

Cognitive Changes

Cognitive changes are common after a stroke, and people who have sustained a stroke may notice changes to their processing ability, thinking and memory, attention, perception, planning ability, social cognition, executive functioning, or ability to communicate. Sometimes the client with stroke will not notice these changes, but their family and friends may notice. These changes may get better after a stroke, and it is uncommon for an individual to experience all of the potential cognitive issues. Changes to cognitive processing can be very frustrating for the person who had the stroke and also to their family and friends. It is important to understand the cognitive changes that may happen after stroke; it will be difficult to use yoga with someone with stroke if you, the therapist, do not understand that the client will need extra time to process information or if they forgot about the left side of their body. Yoga may help improve various aspects of cognitive disability.

Processing

Our brains work hard all day long to process large amounts of information, and this ability to process information may be impacted after a stroke. Changes to how the brain processes the information after a stroke are common. People frequently forget steps to complete common activities. These changes do not mean that a person has dementia, but the changes mean that the client with stroke, and their family, probably will have to do things differently than before the stroke occurred. We have seen people have a lot of trouble differentiating between their right and left sides. This may change how the yoga or rehabilitation therapist delivers yoga as therapy, since people may have a hard time following directions if you tell them to do something with the right arm or leg. Clients with stroke may also need extra time for processing, so the therapists should consider using fewer words and more demonstrations, and allowing time for the client to process information, including verbal directions.

Thinking and Memory

After a stroke, thinking and memory may be compromised; this may mean that your clients with stroke will have a difficult time taking in, storing, and/or retrieving information. There may be changes to both short- and long-term memory, but, after stroke, it is more common that declines in short-term memory are sustained. This may mean that clients with stroke forget appointments, new people who they meet, or where they put an item like glasses or keys. The client may forget things learned in therapy or yoga, and reminders or cues may be necessary. Written reminders may be helpful if the client is able to read.

Attention

The ability to concentrate on something, or maintain attention to something, may be impacted by a stroke. After a stroke, the client may find it quite difficult to know what information to ignore and what information to focus on, making maintaining attention on a task challenging. People with stroke may quickly feel mentally fatigued and may have trouble multitasking. Again, clients with stroke may need extra time to start or complete tasks or movements. The yoga or rehabilitation therapist may want to consider giving one direction at a time or using tactile cues to maintain the client's attention.

Perception

We perceive things by taking in information from the world around us and using our five senses to process the information. Our brain needs to organize all of the incoming information to be able to make sense of it. A stroke may impact the brain's ability to take in this information and organize it. Agnosia is when the brain cannot recognize common objects: the client with stroke may see a toothbrush but not remember what to do with the toothbrush or how to use it. Sometimes after a stroke, people may forget about a side of their body; this is called neglect. Neglect happens because the stroke causes the brain to not process information received from one side of the body. Neglect may happen to either side of the body, but it is more common to have "left neglect" or to neglect or forget about the left side of the body. The severity of the neglect may also be worse on the left side than the right side after a stroke. Left neglect may also be seen when a person with stroke does not eat the food on the left side of the plate. Verbal reminders to move the left arm may or may not work for the client with left neglect. Therefore, the yoga or rehabilitation therapist may need to give tactile or visual cues to remind the client with stroke about the neglected side of the body.

Planning

In therapy, we typically use the word apraxia when talking about challenges with planning movements or actions. Apraxia is a common impairment post-stroke. A person with apraxia may be able to remember what a toothbrush is for but will have trouble actually executing all of the steps of brushing their teeth. For example, the client with stroke may forget to put toothpaste on the toothbrush or to actually brush their teeth. Apraxia of speech may also occur, making it difficult for the client to talk and express themselves. When using yoga for a client with apraxia, consider a physical assist in moving the limb/s through the asana or yoga posture.

Social Cognition

Social cognition is our ability to assess relations between ourselves and others, and to use that information to guide social behavior in future situations. More simply, we use our social cognition to be able to understand and act in different social situations. People with stroke may not be able to engage with others in the way they did before the stroke, they may forget normal social cueing, or they may not be able to show empathy. This may lead to difficulties in relationships after the stroke. Due to the changes in the brain and the enhanced mind-body connection, yoga may allow for improved social cognition over time, even in clients with a chronic stroke.

Executive Functioning

Making decisions is a high-level cognitive skill that may become difficult after a stroke. In therapy, we call this executive functioning and it includes the integration of many of the discussed skills, as well as thinking about all of the information and being able to process it and use it. Executive functioning also includes mental control and self-regulation, so when it is impaired, major challenges may occur for the client with stroke. Initiation, planning, sequencing of steps, and monitoring of directed behaviors are all part of executive functioning. Problem solving may also be more challenging after a stroke if the client has executive functioning issues. Most activities (from basic activities of daily living to driving a car, working, or traveling) will be affected if a stroke limits executive functioning and decision making. When a client has impaired decision-making abilities, it may be best to not ask many questions and not to provide many options to the client. Provide directions through short and direct verbal communication or demonstrate yoga postures or other movements so that the client can follow the movement.

Communication Issues (Aphasia)

Communication is commonly compromised after a stroke; this is called aphasia. Aphasia may occur after a stroke; there are different types of aphasia, and the type and the impact is dependent on where the stroke occurred within the brain. Aphasia impacts the ability to speak and understand what others are saying. The yoga or rehabilitation therapist should remember that aphasia is not a change in intelligence. Depending on the type or severity of the aphasia, the therapist must consider using fewer words for verbal cueing, giving more time to process information, and providing additional time for the client to respond to directions or questions. The use of mantras may be helpful during the yoga practice when clients have a form of aphasia; however, the therapist should be thoughtful about not over stressing the client with mantras at the beginning of their time together.

ANOMIC (OR AMNESIA) APHASIA

Anomic aphasia is considered the least severe type of aphasia. People who have anomic aphasia have trouble using the correct names of objects, places, people, or events. For example, a person with anomic aphasia may see a toothbrush and know what to do with the toothbrush but not know the name of the object.

EXPRESSIVE APHASIA

Expressive aphasia means that the client who has sustained a stroke is not able to find the words to express what they want to, even when they know what they want to say. They have trouble getting information through words or writing out of their head. Often the person may use a few words as their total vocabulary and use those words for all expression. For example, the client may only be able to say "Yep" or "OK" and will use that word for all communication. Sometimes a client may sing the words to the same song over and over again as a response to all questions or conversation.

RECEPTIVE APHASIA

Receptive aphasia means that a client with stroke cannot understand what they are reading or hearing. They have trouble getting information into their brain to be able to process the information. A client with receptive aphasia will have a difficult time following directions in yoga and may do better with mirroring physical movements of the therapist.

GLOBAL APHASIA

While all aphasia is likely frustrating, global aphasia may be the most frustrating for clients with stroke and for their families and friends. It is the most severe type of aphasia and is the combination of expressive and receptive aphasia. Therefore, the client with global aphasia is not able to express themselves, understand speech or directions from others, or read or write.

For all forms of aphasia, it is important to give your clients with stroke short and simple instructions, articulate each word, and give ample time for processing. Additional tips for working with clients with aphasia can be found in Chapter 13.

Emotional Changes

Emotional changes are common after a stroke and often include frustration, anxiety, depression, and emotional regulation (lability). A stroke comes out of nowhere and is typically a shocking and scary event. Clients with stroke may feel many different emotions, not limited to mourning the life they were living, anger, or shock. As for all people, emotions post-stroke will ebb and flow with time, but sometimes after stroke, your client may be more or less emotional than before the stroke. This may be confusing to the client with stroke and to their family and friends; such emotional instability may also limit the client's progress and recovery.

Post-stroke emotional or personality changes may look different for different people and will depend on where in the brain the stroke occurred and their personality prior to the stroke. We know that yoga helps with different emotional and personality changes, including the ability to regulate emotions, so a therapist may consider using yoga for these issues that may arise after a stroke. The Stroke Association of the United Kingdom recommends using mindfulness, meditation, and yoga to stay active and to manage post-stroke emotional changes.

Frustration

Commonly, there is a lot of frustration following a stroke for all involved, including the client with the stroke, their family and friends, and even the yoga or rehabilitation therapist. There may be feelings of shock, worry, grief over lost opportunities or changes in the body, and even guilt about living an unhealthy lifestyle that may have increased the risk of a stroke. A stroke may also limit one's ability to cope with new events or post-stroke changes. The compilation of these emotions may be overwhelming, but this is all fairly common after stroke. It is important to remind the client and the family or friends that changes in cognition, emotions, and physical abilities are common but still frustrating. The buildup of frustrations may make the client with stroke irritable, and they may quickly become angry or frustrated.

Sometimes after a stroke, a client may also be impulsive, making them frustrated more quickly if something doesn't go as expected. Yoga has been shown to help regulate some emotions, such as frustration, or help people with being more OK with their current body or abilities. Additionally, we have found that yoga may improve an individual's ability to cope with new or different issues or people (Crowe, Van Puymbroeck, and Schmid, 2016).

Anxiety

Anxiety is common after a stroke, with about 25% of individuals feeling some level of anxiety during the first five years after the stroke (Campbell Burton, *et al.*, 2013). People may worry about having or causing a future stroke, they may worry about what they cannot do, and they may worry about family and money. They may be worried about falling or develop a fear of falling or of moving and hurting themselves (Schmid, *et al.*, 2009, 2015a). Yoga may help to reduce anxiety and fear, while at the same time improving things like balance or strength to reduce the actual risk of a fall or pain during movement. In our research we continually find improvements in fear of falling, also thought of as falls efficacy, or the confidence to not fall or lose balance (balance self-efficacy or balance confidence) (Schmid, Van Puymbroeck, and Koceja, 2010; Schmid, *et al.*, 2012; Van Puymbroeck, *et al.*, 2017). We most often measure anxiety with the Generalized Anxiety Disorder Scale. We have not found significant improvements in generalized anxiety for clients with stroke who complete yoga with us; however, people who agree to be in an eight-week yoga study tend to not be very anxious. Other researchers who focus on anxiety and include people with increased levels of anxiety do consistently demonstrate that yoga improves anxiety (Kirkwood, *et al.*, 2005). For clients with stroke who also have higher levels of anxiety, we suspect that yoga will be of benefit in managing their anxiety.

Depression

Depression may develop after a stroke, and the depression may be due to the fact that the client had the stroke and may feel sad about the occurrence of the stroke or loss of abilities. However, depression may also occur due to neurological changes that occur in the brain related to the stroke. It is thought that approximately 33% of people who sustain a stroke will develop some level of depression (commonly called post-stroke depression or PSD) (Paolucci, 2008). Depression will impact recovery and potentially limit the influence of therapy and adherence to home exercise programs. We most often use the Patient Health Questionnaire as our depression outcome measure. Some clients will require anti-depressants, medications that may help alleviate the signs and symptoms of post-stroke depression. A medical doctor must be involved in the diagnosis and pharmaceutical treatment of both anxiety and depression, but clinicians and therapists must be aware of the diagnosis and the effects of both the diagnosis and the side effects of the medications. Medications do not cure emotional issues such as depression or anxiety, but medications may help to make things feel better or easier. The impact of yoga on post-stroke depression has not been studied; however, a review of the literature indicates that yoga is beneficial in the management of depression (Cramer, *et al.*, 2013)—thus yoga is likely to also help improve post-stroke depression.

Emotional Regulation or Lability

Commonly, people with stroke will have difficulties with regulating emotions. This may also be called emotionalism or emotional lability (being labile). Emotions may feel out of control and these emotions can cycle very quickly. A person may be overly emotional and become upset very easily, or very happy over little things, at a magnitude not necessarily appropriate for the situation. A person may cry for no reason and some people become embarrassed by their new post-stroke emotions. Some emotional regulation changes may be related to post-stroke depression but may also be a symptom of stroke. In a small study, we found that yoga improves emotional regulation in people with traumatic brain injury, and stroke is a type of brain injury (Grimm, *et al.*, 2017). Thus, when you use yoga for a client with stroke who has challenges with emotional regulation, the client may tell you they are noticing changes or improvements in their emotions—often people talk about crying less or feeling more like their old self from before the stroke. Equanimity is a term used frequently in yoga and is the idea of having mental calmness and being able to maintain the calmness even during stressful or difficult times. Being able to maintain composure may be related to emotional regulation, and equanimity is also thought to be enhanced through yoga. Yoga may help with emotional regulation or equanimity, as it is thought that as the mind calms, the body will follow.

Physical Changes

Post-stroke physical changes vary greatly in scope and severity and include changes in both sensation or sensory (feeling) and motor (moving) capabilities. There may be post-stroke changes involving: proprioception (knowing where the body is in space); hemiparesis; muscle weakness; dysarthria; foot drop; asymmetry; fatigue; spasticity; vision; pain; and fall-related issues such as balance, strength, and range of motion. As a client with stroke becomes physically or mentally fatigued, other cognitive, emotional, or physical challenges may become more apparent or appear to become more severe. It is important for the therapist who is using yoga as therapy to be able to monitor fatigue and other physiological changes to best gauge therapy intensity and duration, maintaining safety for the client. Monitoring blood pressure and oxygen saturation may provide information related to physiological changes in the client; see Chapter 14 for additional information on monitoring these physiological responses to yoga.

Sensory and Motor Changes

Many clients sustain changes in sensory or sensation after a stroke—thus a client may not be able to feel their arm or their leg. Proprioception, or knowing where one's body is in space, may also be decreased after a stroke. A loss of proprioception may mean the client will have difficulties moving the limb as they wish and they may often have to look at the limb to know where the arm or the leg is in space. Additionally, the client may feel as if the limb does not belong to them or that the limb has somehow changed in shape or size. Encouraging the client to bear weight in the limb with decreased sensation or proprioception is thought to help provide the nervous system with helpful feedback. Table Top (Goasana) or Cat Cow (Chakravakasana) (see Chapter 6) may provide such stimulation if the client can tolerate being in quadruped (bearing weight on all fours).

Change in sensation after stroke may mean less or more sensation than normal or before the stroke. It is common that, after a client sustains a stroke, they will have less ability to sense being touched. The client may not be able to feel pressure or pain and therefore be at risk for injury. The client may also not be able to feel temperatures and consequently be at risk for burns. Some clients with stroke will actually have increased sensation, called hyperesthesia. This is not limited to just touch but may be a hyperawareness of sound, smell, or taste. When integrating yoga into rehabilitation, it is important for the yoga or rehabilitation therapist to ask about sensation sensitivity and what the client can feel or not feel, and whether noises or smells may be bothersome or distracting. Using music or essential oils may distract a client with sensory issues; however, the therapist may consider adding in such sensory stimulants over time.

HEMIPARESIS OR WEAKNESS

After sustaining a stroke, it is common for the client to have muscle weakness; in fact up to 75% of people who have sustained a stroke have weakness after a stroke (Management of Stroke Rehabilitation Working Group, 2010). The weakness may in fact be paralysis, meaning that the client is not able to feel or move the limb that is paralyzed, commonly referred to as paretic. The paralysis may be considered "dense," meaning the client has little to no sensation or movement. However, the paralysis may also not be "dense" but somewhere in the middle between "dense" and "normal." After a stroke, related to its location and severity, it is common that the client will be paralyzed on half of the body—the left arm and left leg or the right arm and right leg; this is referred to as hemiparesis (hemi means "half"). Interestingly, if a stroke occurs on the right side of the brain, the person may experience left-sided symptoms, while right-sided symptoms will occur after a stroke that occurs on the left side of the brain.

When a client has hemiparesis, they may have challenges in activities of daily living as well as balance and mobility, placing them at greater risk for falls. It is important for the yoga or rehabilitation therapist to remember that sensation may be compromised and that the therapist may injure the client but the client will not be able to feel pain. Through our yoga studies, we have found that some clients actually benefit with improved sensation; for example, we have heard more than one client say in a surprised voice, "I can feel my foot!" Additionally, and more commonly, we have found great improvements in motor control, meaning the client is more able to move the limb in a controlled fashion than before the yoga intervention. We often see this manifest with movement in the feet or the hands and then the improved sensation or the improved movement moves more proximally, or towards the core center of the body. While not truly understood, the sense of the mind and body reconnecting with yoga may be associated with improved awareness of afferent (sensory) feedback, allowing for more effective efferent (motor) commands to muscles.

DYSARTHRIA

Dysarthria is related to speaking and communication but is secondary to decreases in motor capabilities after a stroke—not the processing of words or information. It is the decreased ability to control the muscles of the face, mouth, and the throat needed for speech. Dysarthria may become evident as challenges with: articulation or pronunciation of words; how loud a person may be able to speak; and how fast a person can speak words. When a client has dysarthria, provide them with enough time to speak. Some postures, such as Lion's pose (Simhasana) (see Chapter 6), may help to strengthen the muscles of the face, mouth, and throat that are impacted by dysarthria. Short mantras that can easily be repeated may also be helpful (see Chapters 5 and 12).

FOOT DROP

After a stroke, clients who have a foot drop may require the use of an ankle foot orthosis, which is a brace that maintains the ankle and foot in proper positioning to reduce the risk of tripping or falling. The yoga or rehabilitation therapist may need to take off the ankle foot orthosis to best provide therapy and stimulate movement, but the therapist must correctly replace it prior to the end of therapy. If the ankle foot orthosis is not on correctly, and the client has decreased sensation, there is a risk the client may develop a wound, which may limit recovery and, in some circumstances, may lead to hospitalization or even death. Therefore, if the therapist does not feel confident in correctly replacing the orthosis, they should consider leaving it on during yoga. This is true of any brace or orthosis after a stroke. The therapist should remember that the client is required to don and doff any brace or orthosis on a daily basis. Therefore, depending on the client, the therapist may also rely on the client to correctly and safely manage the orthosis.

ASYMMETRY AFTER A STROKE

Asymmetry is common after a stroke; this means that the body, or even the face, may be asymmetrical as a result of the stroke. The asymmetry may be related to a lack of sensory input to the muscles or the inability to control the muscles (changes in sensory or motor abilities). It is common in rehabilitation practice to, as possible and as tolerated, move the client into quadruped (weight bearing on all fours). This is also true for yoga after a stroke; the therapist may consider including Table Top (Goasana) or Cat Cow (Chakravakasana) (see Chapter 6) to help improve post-stroke asymmetry.

When the client cannot get to the floor, consider using a fold-down mat table or stationary mat table. Moving into prone postures is challenging and should most often be reserved for one-to-one practices when the therapist can manage the needs of the client.

FATIGUE

We have found that fatigue is common after a stroke and that it is related to pain (Miller, et al., 2013). Both fatigue and pain negatively impact other aspects of function, as well as recovery. It appears that post-stroke fatigue is not well studied or understood. However, after working with many clients with stroke, it is clear that post-stroke fatigue is different than just being tired. Napping and sleeping do not seem to fully manage or improve post-stroke fatigue. We believe it is important for the client with stroke, the therapist, and the family to understand that post-stroke fatigue is not the client being "lazy" and cannot be corrected by taking a nap. Post-stroke fatigue may never fully go away, but it seems helpful when everyone understands this concept. Indeed, we have worked with clients who sustained their stroke a decade ago, and we commonly hear the same comments about fatigue. Fatigue is not only physical; it may also be mental or emotional fatigue. Being more physically active, perhaps through yoga, may help manage fatigue by improving cardiovascular fitness, including blood flow to both sides of the brain.

It does appear that yoga may help with physical fatigue after a stroke (Lazaridou, Philbrook, and Tzika, 2013); we also believe yoga may help with the client being more in the moment and being more content. Being a bit more content may help the client, and the family, from over scheduling other activities. Occupational therapists might help to address fatigue through effective energy-conservation techniques. But we also encourage the yoga or rehabilitation therapist to consider using restorative postures in the yoga practice, or as part of a home exercise program. Through the use of restorative yoga practices, it may be possible to calm and quiet the nervous system, allowing it to better recover. See Chapter 7 for restorative poses to be used after stroke to quiet the nervous system and allow the body to relax.

SPASTICITY

It is common for clients with stroke to have some spasticity, which means that the muscles are very tight due to increased tone or constant muscle contraction. In individuals post-stroke, it is common to see an arm in spasticity, with a very flexed wrist and elbow and sometimes a shoulder that is internally rotated. Spasticity occurs because the neurological messages from the brain to the muscles are not being transmitted through the nerves as they did prior to the stroke. The muscle then begins to contract and cannot stop contracting, resulting in interference with normal muscle movements or movement patterns. It is important to manage spasticity through stretching and perhaps through splinting. Splinting is often completed by the occupational therapist in the hopes of maintaining maximum range of motion at a joint. If the spasticity is not managed well, a contracture may develop. A contracture is the permanent shortening of the muscles, meaning the joint becomes stuck and the muscles and joint cannot be fully stretched to their full length (a straight or extended elbow and wrist). Range of motion is commonly limited after a stroke but becomes even more limited once a contracture develops. Spasticity must be managed during the acute recovery phase of the stroke to prevent contractures from developing. Yoga may be used to stretch the muscles and maintain proper positioning. In the client with a more chronic stroke who has developed a contracture, the therapist must be very cautious to not cause any pain or injury to the joint or muscles by stretching the muscles too far. The yoga or rehabilitation therapist should also remember that if there is a lack of or decreased sensation, the client may not be able to feel or sense when an injury is occurring (see Chapter 14 for strategies to prevent injuries).

VISION CHANGES AND VISUAL FIELD CUTS

Changes in vision are common but complicated after a stroke. Approximately a third of people who sustain a stroke experience some change to their vision (Stroke Foundation, 2018). The types of visual changes that occur after a stroke cannot be corrected through glasses. It is common that vision in both eyes will be impacted after stroke, because the nerves from each eye travel together in the brain. Additionally, if there is damage to one side of the brain (let's consider the right side of the brain), the left-sided vision will be impacted in *both* eyes (see Figure 2.1). The actual movement of the eye may also be compromised secondary to nerve damage after the stroke. This damage may cause the eye muscle to stop working or to work incorrectly, potentially leading to diplopia or double vision.

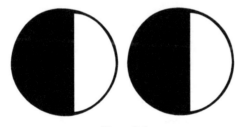

Figure 2.1

The visual field may be altered after a stroke. The "visual field" is the broad area that the eye sees when the eye is in a fixed position. If there is a field cut, it is likely that both eyes are affected. If a client has homonymous hemianopia, they will only be able to see half of what they are looking at. For example, if they cannot see the left visual field, the client will not be able to see the left side of words on a page or will not be able to see the left side of a face. The therapist must take this into account when providing written or video recordings of home exercise programs. A client may also develop quadrantanopia after the stroke and may not be able to see the upper or lower quadrant of the visual field in both eyes.

Yoga may help the client with post-stroke vision changes; consider including the yoga eye exercises described in Chapter 5. Also, when appropriate, encourage the client to visually track the movement of the limb through space when completing yoga postures.

PAIN

Pain is common but complex after a stroke. Because there may be both motor and sensory changes, the sensation of pain may also be compromised. Clients who have limited or no sensation may not feel pain when they should and may be more likely to sustain injuries. It is not surprising for a client to get a hemiparetic hand "stuck" in the spokes of the wheelchair, simply because they cannot feel the pain (and may not recognize where their hand is in space due to other changes in sensation or perception). Despite the lack of pain, or maybe because of it, clients with stroke may be at higher risk for sustaining an injury. The therapist must therefore not rely on the client to indicate pain and must be cautious to not cause injury during yoga or other aspects of therapy. For some clients with post-stroke changes in sensation, pain may include unusual sensations, such as tingling, cold, or burning. For clients with motor functioning changes, there may be pain related to spasticity or stiffness. It is common for clients after a stroke to have pain in the shoulder or have a subluxed shoulder (when the shoulder is weak and allows for the humeral head to move out of the glenoid cavity of the shoulder). Additionally, clients with stroke commonly report headaches. In our studies we have found that pain intensity or severity does not always change for clients but the impact of pain on function or day-to-day life does improve with yoga. Once a client in a study told us, "Yoga didn't really change the pain, it [yoga] just helped me put the pain somewhere else, and [I was] not always thinking about it."

INCREASED FALL RISKS: BALANCE, STRENGTH, AND RANGE OF MOTION

After a stroke, clients have a substantially increased likelihood of falling (Forster and Young, 1995; Schmid, et al., 2013a). We have found that 76% of people with stroke report that they sustained at least one fall sometime after the occurrence of the stroke (Schmid, et al., 2013a). Falls after a stroke are linked to the development of fear of falling, worse functional outcomes, increased fracture rates, and even death, and therefore it is important that fall prevention be addressed during therapy.

There are many fall risk factors (or things that make falls more likely) following a stroke; many have already been discussed, including: changes in sensation; hemiparesis; asymmetry; fatigue; spasticity; visual changes; and pain. Changes in balance, strength, and range of motion (flexibility) are also important fall risk factors and are each commonly challenged after stroke. Much of our yoga research has focused on decreasing fall rates through improving balance and other fall risk factors.

Because of primary damage in the central brain structures, and secondary effects on sensory and physical systems, balance is commonly compromised after stroke. It is known that balance is complex, as it necessitates the integration of the brain working with multiple body systems (Rogers and Martinez, 2009). Muscle strength and range of motion are also required for balance and are often decreased after a stroke, as already discussed in the sections about hemiparesis and spasticity. Balance deficits are related to poor recovery of activities of daily living, worse functional mobility, and increased fall risks (Management of Stroke Rehabilitation Working Group, 2010). Balance impairment is also directly linked to decreased quality of life, and thus improving balance may give the client the opportunity to also improve their quality of life (Schmid, *et al.*, 2013a).

Our completed research studies support that yoga improves balance after stroke and that the improvement in balance is likely related to improved lower extremity strength and range of motion, but also improved proprioception and confidence. We provide more information about stroke and yoga research studies in Chapter 4. Additionally, we provide evidence-based sample practices from our research in Chapter 12 and include a practice that we have found to improve post-stroke balance for clients with chronic stroke. We most commonly use the Berg Balance Scale (Berg, Wood-Dauphinee, and Williams, 1995), a physical performance test, to assess balance. The Berg Balance Scale includes 14 items that assess static and dynamic balance. Examples of assessment items that measure static balance include: standing unsupported for up to two minutes; sitting unsupported in a chair for two minutes; and tandem standing (one foot in front of the other, toe to heal) for up to 30 seconds. There are additional items that assess dynamic balance (to maintain balance while in motion) and include: transferring or moving from one chair to another chair (or bed); bending over and picking up an object from the floor; turning 360 degrees; and stepping each foot on and off of a step stool.

The yoga or rehabilitation therapist may choose to challenge the client's balance once the therapist feels comfortable and confident in doing so with each individual client. Both sitting and standing postures will likely lead to improved balance. In addition, the use of a chair or the wall will facilitate the inclusion of standing practices. Among other poses, Warrior I (Virabhadrasana I) or Crescent Lunge (Anjeneyasana) may challenge balance while simultaneously improving flexibility and strength to the lower extremity muscles and joints.

Decreased Overall Function and Quality of Life Are Common After a Stroke

Due to the collective challenges and changes in cognitive, emotional, and physical abilities after a stroke, it is common to see decreases in overall functioning and quality of life. For example, clients with stroke commonly have decreased mobility, which is complex and comprised of numerous systems working together and allowing for sensation, motor control, balance, strength, range of motion, flexibility, perception, and processing to work together. Activities of daily living and instrumental activities of daily living are also commonly challenged after a stroke. Activities of daily living include basic daily living skills, such as dressing, bathing, hygiene, and eating—the things we each do every day to get out of the house and on with our days. Instrumental activities of daily living are a bit more complex and include cooking, planning meals, home management, banking, shopping, and other higher-level activities that may require leaving the home.

Because yoga has numerous benefits and seems to improve many cognitive, emotional, and physical outcomes, it also seems to be associated with improvements in mobility, activities of daily living, and instrumental activities of daily living. We have found improvements in endurance and walking speed, as well as improvements in daily living skills. Overall, clients with chronic stroke have shown improvements in overall function and quality of life after eight weeks of group yoga (Schmid, *et al.*, 2012, 2014). For example:

> One woman, named Addya (a pseudonym), completed one of our yoga research studies after her stroke. She received 16 one-hour sessions of yoga over eight weeks. She then told us about life-changing improvements in her mobility and activities of daily living, allowing her to greatly enhance her day-to-day life and participate more fully in activities that made her content and happy. Addya, and the research team, teared up as she told her powerful story about her life after yoga...
>
> Addya had sustained a stroke over ten years ago, and while she lived independently at home, she had many limitations and stroke-related disability. Addya shared with us that, while she was happy to live at home, she was not able to successfully complete many of her activities of daily living after she sustained her stroke. Most significantly, she told us that she was not very easily able to safely shower or bathe after her stroke. She was afraid to fall while in the shower and had trouble getting in and out of the shower or bath tub. Due to her concerns about her safety, Addya did not frequently shower, and unfortunately then stopped seeing her friends and engaging in activities due to her lack of hygiene. Addya told us that she was embarrassed by her lack of hygiene, and her subsequent odor; she really stopped living her life outside of her home and she became isolated. Within weeks of her practicing yoga as part of our study, Addya noticed improved balance, strength, range of motion, and even improved balance confidence. She felt less depressed and more in control of her mind and body. She shared with us that she was again able to successfully and safely shower! Her new ability to shower and her change in hygiene gave Addya the momentum and confidence she needed to reconnect with her friends and to start going out into her community. She said, "I was able to shower again, and you cannot believe how much that means to me!" She was also able to return to activities she had not done since before her stroke. Addya reminded us of the power of yoga to be life changing, and for her it truly was!

Location, Location, Location

Stroke-related disability is common after a stroke and may include cognitive, emotional, and physical changes after the stroke. The location of the stroke and the side of the brain where the stroke occurred matter and are related to the disability that is evident post-stroke. Depending on the location of the stroke and the residual disability, each person with stroke presents differently and should be treated as a unique individual; the use of a client-centered, or individual, approach is recommended.

If the stroke occurred on the *left* side of the brain, the person with stroke is more likely to demonstrate:

- motor and sensory impairment to the right side of the body and/or face

- speech or language impairment

- slow, cautious, or obsessive decision making or behaviors

- memory loss

- apraxia or impaired motor control (getting the body to do what the brain wants)

- aphasia or challenges with speaking (expressive aphasia) or understanding speech (receptive aphasia).

People who have a stroke on the *right* side of the brain are more likely to have:

- motor and sensory impairment to the left side of the body and/or face

- vision impairments

- emotional lability or extreme high and low emotions that might include involuntary laughing or crying

- change in memory or memory loss

- short attention spans

- loss of concentration

- impulsive or impaired decision making or behaviors

- spatial-perceptual loss; they may have left neglect.

After a stroke to the *brain stem*, people might have:

- motor and sensory impairment to both the left and right of the body. This results in no movement below the neck and being "locked in" to the body.

Who Makes Up the Post-Stroke Team?

The post-stroke team is made up of many clinicians and therapists, many of whom may use yoga as a part of treatment to enhance recovery and healing. Here, we discuss some of the most commonly included team members.

The Client with Stroke and Their Family and Loved Ones Are Part of the Team

The most important member of the team is really the individual who has sustained the stroke! When treating the individual with stroke, their interests, abilities, and goals should be discussed to determine treatment plans. Therefore, when choosing treatment interventions, such as yoga, the client and their family should be involved. Yoga may not be for everyone, or sometimes an individual is not quite ready to try yoga. See Chapter 13 for tips on introducing yoga to new clients with stroke.

Occupational Therapists

Occupational therapists use occupation, or meaningful activity, to promote health, well-being, and recovery. Occupational therapists are concerned about how clients occupy their time and, when working with people with stroke, will often focus on helping the client to engage in old or new occupations. Occupational therapists utilize a holistic approach, meaning they emphasize treating the whole person, mind, body, and spirit. Therefore, from what we hear, a lot of occupational therapists have begun to use yoga in their clinical practice. For some clients, yoga may even become a new occupation or activity that they enjoy after their stroke rehabilitation has ended.

For additional information about occupational therapy, check out these websites:

- Royal College of Occupational Therapists: www.rcot.co.uk

- American Occupational Therapy Association: www.aota.org

- World Federation of Occupational Therapists: www.wfot.org.

Recreational Therapists

Recreational therapists use recreation and leisure activities to improve function and well-being in individuals with acute or chronic disease and disability. In a rehabilitation setting, recreational therapists would use a recreation activity that is enjoyable to the client to target the affected area of the body. Recreational therapists aim to help people return to their enjoyable activities. Many recreational therapists are incorporating yoga into their practice because yoga, like recreational therapy, is holistic and enhances the mind-body connection.

For additional information about recreation therapy, check out this website:

- American Therapeutic Recreation Association: www.atra-online.com.

Physios or Physical Therapists

Physical therapists help people to reduce pain and improve mobility to allow achievement of long-term health benefits. After stroke, physical therapy is commonly focused on improving balance, strength, and range of motion in the lower extremities to allow for improvements related to gait and mobility.

For additional information about physio or physical therapy, check out these websites:

- Chartered Society of Physiotherapy: www.csp.org.uk

- American Physical Therapy Association: www.apta.org

- World Confederation for Physical Therapy: www.wcpt.org.

Speech Language Pathologists

Speech language pathologists work with individuals who have difficulty with communication, cognitive issues, and swallowing disorders. After a stroke, language disorders may occur, and the speech language pathologist can help to target receptive and expressive language difficulties. The speech language pathologist may also assist with identifying and treating swallowing disorders that occur after stroke.

For additional information about speech language pathologists, check out these websites:

- Royal College of Speech and Language Therapists: www.rcslt.org

- American Speech-Language-Hearing Association: www.asha.org

- International Association of Logopedics and Phoniatrics: www.ialp.info.

Stroke Neurologists

A neurologist is a medical doctor who specializes in disorders and treatments of the brain and the nervous system. A stroke neurologist is one who specializes in the treatment of stroke and commonly works closely with the client, the family, and the nursing and rehabilitation team. The stroke neurologist may be involved with the client from when the client arrives in the Emergency Department, through the entire trajectory of stroke care. Check out additional information from this website:

- American Stroke Association: www.strokeassociation.org/STROKEORG.

Yoga Therapists

Yoga therapists have extensive training in using yoga in a clinical and therapeutic practice. Yoga may be used to treat different aspects of stroke. The mission of the International Association of Yoga Therapists "is to establish yoga as a recognized and respected therapy." Yoga therapists consider all aspects of yoga as therapy. Other therapists who are part of the post-stroke team are more likely to use yoga as part of therapy, as an occupation, as a leisure activity, or as a modality that is included as part of therapy.

For additional information about yoga therapy, check out this international website:

- International Association of Yoga Therapists: www.iayt.org.

Summary

In summary, strokes are complex and may lead to many post-stroke disabilities and challenges for the client. Each individual with stroke will present differently and will have different needs. Secondary to neuroplasticity, change and recovery may happen after a stroke and a yoga intervention may lead to improvements in cognitive, emotional, and physical improvements. Yoga, and its philosophical underpinnings, are further explored in Chapter 3.

Exploring Yoga Basics

A HOLISTIC APPROACH TO THERAPY AFTER STROKE

As discussed in Chapter 2 in the review of stroke and stroke interventions, a stroke impacts the whole person, not just the physical body. Yoga is an intervention that treats the whole person and therefore addresses the emotional, cognitive, and physical changes that may occur after stroke. This chapter includes a comprehensive summary of yoga philosophy and will likely be a review for yoga therapists and yoga teachers. Rehabilitation therapists who are integrating yoga into practice may be doing so because they have learned about yoga and personally practice yoga. However, they may not have advanced training in yoga and yogic philosophy. This chapter offers information about yoga and suggestions of using yoga for clients with stroke.

Eastern and Western medicine address the body and impairments differently. While Eastern philosophies are more holistic and work towards health and well-being, Western medicine typically focuses on the disease or on the physical body and often forgets about emotional and cognitive influences as complicating factors in health. Stress and worry, including negative self-talk, may impede healing and recovery but are less often addressed in Western medicine. This may be slowly changing as more Western medical schools are beginning to add course work on the benefits of integrative medicine and therapies, such as yoga and recovery after a stroke. Yogic practices are of Eastern descent, specifically from India, and treat the whole person.

Each author has completed a yoga teacher training in different traditions; however, regardless of the type of yoga (i.e. Hatha yoga, Lakshmi Voelker chair yoga, Kundalini yoga, or Viniyoga), all yoga teachers should receive training and education about the same fundamentals of yoga, including the Yoga Sutras of Patanjali. Here we briefly review the underpinnings of yogic philosophies and how yoga may influence health and wellness and recovery after stroke. Arlene completed her yoga teacher training with River Cummings and brilliant yoga therapists in Fort Collins, CO. All of her yoga philosophy course content was taught by Michael Lloyd-Billington (2014). Please see writings offered by Michael for additional information regarding yogic philosophies. Michael teaches yogic philosophies in many different yoga teacher trainings in Fort Collins, CO, United States (www.thelivingyogablog.com).

When using yoga to treat clients with stroke, it is essential to know the client as an individual and develop the yoga intervention in a client-centered way, which best meets the needs of that person. Yoga in rehabilitation after a stroke may look different for an occupational, physical, or recreational therapist who is using yoga as a part of rehabilitation treatment in a hospital or very clinical setting, versus a yoga therapist who is comprehensively using yoga as the full treatment intervention in a hospital or rehabilitation setting, a yoga studio, or a community-based setting. Regardless, it is important to understand the underpinnings of yoga and how yoga can alter the therapeutic process for clients with stroke.

Everyone Can Do Yoga

It is our belief, gained through our own personal yoga practices, using yoga with clients, and our research studies, that as long as a person can follow instructions and can breathe independently, they can engage in a practice of yoga. We also believe that a person with a tracheostomy who cannot breathe on their own can likely still practice mindfulness, meditation, and potentially some asanas. Individuals with very limited movement or independent breathing can also utilize mental practice to receive a number of the benefits outlined in Chapter 5. Mental practice, or the idea of thinking about moving a limb through a posture or moving fingers through mudras, may also lead to improvements. Research studies by Dr. Stephen Page and his research team (Page, *et al.*, 2001; Page, Levine, and Leonard, 2007) provide evidence that supports the idea of encouraging mental practice after stroke; mental practice of performing specific yoga asanas may enhance neural pathways. In our studies with people with stroke, clients are always encouraged to imagine their limb or fingers moving to match the movement of the other limb. Mental practice should be encouraged for all phases of stroke recovery and allows all clients with stroke to do yoga and increase neural recovery. Mental practice is also safe and can be performed independently without a therapist's supervision, so it's a great part of a home exercise program!

What Is Yoga?

Yoga is an ancient practice from India, dating back 5000 years. The word yoga means to "union," "yoke," or unite. At its most basic, yoga is a practice that engages the whole person, including the mind, body, and soul. This suggests that the whole person (mind, body, and spirit) is united through yoga.

Background
Western Medicine

According to Hippocrates (born 460 BC), a Greek physician and the father of medicine (think Hippocratic oath), the body has within it anything and everything it needs to heal and recover. His therapeutic approach to medicine and therapy, based on nature and treating the whole person, was lost when Europe slipped into the dark ages. As time progressed, the thought that there was a split between the mind and the body deepened; this was true for both diagnoses and treatment. Soon, it was thought that illness was only a physical phenomenon and that disease and treatment did not have any impact on the mind or soul. In the 1600s, René Descartes further delineated the mind (consciousness and self-awareness) from the brain (intelligence), broadening the idea that the mind and body are not connected. Mental health disability was treated through the use of harsh punishments and restraints. Not until mental illness was correlated to physiological changes in the brain were mental health interventions developed and studied. Finally, it was understood that other diseases of the body also have origins in the mind. Slowly, it is becoming recommended that the best interventions must treat the mind and body together, not separately.

Ayurvedic Medicine

In contrast to Western medicine, Ayurveda is a traditional system of Indian medicine and considered to be one of the oldest holistic approaches to healing. The English translation of the word Ayurvedic is life (ayur) and knowledge (veda) (life knowledge). Ayurvedic practitioners indicate that health and wellness, and recovery from illness, consist of a necessary balance between the mind, the body, and the spirit. Ayurveda and yoga are not the same, but they are related. For example, both Ayurvedic medicine and yoga date back over 5000 years, are derived from a greater system of Vedic knowledge, and are used as holistic treatments. Both consist of or include: doshas or energies; subtle channels (nadis); eight branches or limbs of practice; sheaths (koshas); and energy centers (chakras). Yoga may be used to treat some of the imbalances addressed through Ayurvedic medicine.

Yogic Philosophies
The Doshas

In Ayurvedic medicine, there are three doshas or energies and yoga may be used to balance the doshas, or the basic constitution of each of us. The three doshas are vata, pitta, and kapha, and each of us is made up of a combination of each of the doshas. We do each have a primary dosha that rules our mood, energy, and health. The doshas are influenced by the environment, diet, seasons, climate, age, and other factors, and the doshas may go in and out of balance. The balance of the doshas is said to influence our moods, energy, and health in general; in essence the doshas are the blueprint or our prakriti (nature). Yoga is said to balance the doshas. See Table 3.1 for information about each of the doshas.

Table 3.1: Information about the three doshas

Dosha	Element	Characterized by	Other information	Ailments associated with imbalance	Asana and pranayama for balancing the dosha
Vata dosha	Air	Dry, cold, light, movement	All body movement is due to vata	Pain, flatulence, gout, arthritis, muscle wasting, fractures	• Standing Forward Bend (Uttanasana) • Child's pose (Balasana) • Corpse pose (Savasana) • Alternate Nostril Breathing (Nadi Shodhana Pranayama)
Pitta dosha	Fire (mostly) and water	Hot, moist, liquid, sharp, sour	Heat and energy	Digestive issues, heartburn, acid reflux, nausea, diarrhea	• Cobra pose (Bhujangasana) • Locust pose (Salabhasana) • Cooling Breath (Sitali Pranayama)
Kapha dosha	Water and earth (to make mud)	Cold, heaviness, softness, slowness, the carrier of nutrients	Organs are made of kapha, kapha nourishes and lubricates joints	Varicose veins and thrombosis, hardening of the blood vessels, high cholesterol, swelling, obesity	• Standing poses, such as Tree pose (Vrksasana), Warrior II (Virabhadrasana II), Twisting Chair pose (Parivrtta Utkatasana) • Bridge pose (Setu Bandha Sarvangasana) • Breath of Fire/ Skull Shining Breath (Kapalabhati Pranayama) • Bellows Breath (Bhastrika Pranayama)

The Yoga Sutras of Patanjali

The Yoga Sutras is one of the great ancient texts of yoga and consists of 196 sutras (or "threads" in Sanskrit). Patanjali is considered the father of modern yoga and he wrote the Yoga Sutras in about 400 CE. The Yoga Sutras are considered a collection of aphorisms, or sayings, that are a pathway to a meaningful and purposeful life. It should be noted that while the Yoga Sutras are a pathway to a meaningful and purposeful life, the Yoga Sutras do not include information or direction for expert or perfected poses or alignment. Where possible we do however include yoga postures, pranayama, or mantras for therapists to consider when working with clients with stroke.

The Nadis

In the most basic sense, the nadis are the channels in all of us in which the energies (or prana) of the physical body, subtle body, and causal body flow. The nadis are described differently in different yogic texts, but most agree that the nadis carry the life force, or the prana. Therefore, it is thought that breath work, or pranayama, influences the nadis. Most agree that there may be thousands of channels for the energy to flow, but in some traditions, there may be three main channels or pathways. These three nadis run through the body—one to the left of the spine (ida), one to the right of the spine (pingala), and one through the center of the spinal cord, through the seven chakras (sushumna; see under "The Chakras" later in this chapter). Ida has a cooling effect and courses through the left side of the body, is governed by the right hemisphere of the brain, and controls all mental processes. Pingala is warming in nature and moves along the right side of the body, controls the vital processes of the body, and corresponds to the left hemisphere of the brain. Remember that the left hemisphere of the brain controls the motor and sensory systems of the right side of the body, and vice versa. Breath work, or pranayama, is used in yoga to influence the flow of the prana through the nadis. We include Alternate Nostril Breathing (Nadi Shodhana Pranayama) (see Chapter 8) in all of our yoga research studies, as it may activate both hemispheres of the brain.

The Five Obstacles

Patanjali identified the five kleshas or obstacles that we all face and that are always with us and with our clients. The kleshas are the obstacles, or the veils, to finding our internal peace or to being whole, with the mind and the body connected. Perhaps, after stroke, the kleshas are also the obstacles to recovery and progress. When using yoga for therapy after stroke, it is important to recognize the five kleshas and how the obstacles may be standing in the way of the client's progress and recovery. It is believed that any form of disease or discomfort can be traced back to one or a combination of the five kleshas. The practice of yoga helps to manage the things that obstruct our experiences; it takes connection of the mind and body to truly remove or manage the obstacles. Once the obstacles are understood, then yoga may be used to manage the obstacles, which are listed here.

- **Avidya: ignorance or false knowledge**. Patanjali tells us that avidya is the foundation of the other kleshas, meaning that all the other kleshas may be traced back to misunderstandings or misperceptions. Under avidya, there are two categories. The first category is to hold a belief that is not accurate or true. The second category is the lack of knowledge or awareness. Here, ignorance is not necessarily a lack of education or knowledge, but it is our lack of awareness or the inability to see the truth. Avidya may be a disconnect from the truth, but the lack of truth, knowledge, or awareness can be as painful or challenging as falsehoods or lies. This disconnect from the truth after a stroke may be related to recovery, efforts required for recovery, or simply a lack of awareness of the post-stroke disability that may have occurred. The enhancement of the mind and body connection that occurs with yoga may help people to come to a truth or awareness of their post-stroke abilities and be more content with the changes and the recovery since the occurrence of the stroke.

- **Asmita: over identifying with your ego or egoism, our transcendental self.** Well, we all have an ego! Our ego is essential and necessary as we develop and grow and become the people we are to become. Our ego may be the way we label ourselves or think of ourselves. And our ego often gets in the way or gets us into trouble; our ego may allow us to distort reality. This is not any different for clients with stroke who are using yoga as therapy, as ego is partly how we view ourselves and view the people around us. After a stroke, an individual may already have a skewed view of themselves or of their abilities. Yoga may help alter the client's perception and help them to not compare and contrast themselves to their prior self or to others with stroke.

- **Raga: attachment, desire, or attachment to pleasure.** We all need or want things. Things may be people, a loved one, a pet, an object, or the newest and greatest thing. However, in yogic philosophy, it is not healthy to be overly attached to wanting something or to the actual things. It is thought that such obsession or focus on something obstructs our overall view of life. We often see this in yoga when people become very attached to being able to successfully complete a certain challenging pose. When we are overly attached to a thing or an idea we can hurt ourselves or become less healthy. After a stroke, we find that people are often very attached to who they used to be or who they *think* they used to be. After a stroke, our clients can become obsessed with the recovery of an ability, of a movement, or of the ability to speak in the same way again. The truth is that the very specific ability they so desire may never happen again during their recovery, but being too attached to that one piece of progress may prevent them from making progress in their unique recovery path. We know that when people are so attached to who they once were, they have a hard time becoming the new person they are meant to be after their stroke. After years of researching yoga for people with stroke, we have seen that once people can be in the moment and accept where and who they are, they can move forward to their recovery. We know that yoga helps to manage some of the negative self-talk that we all do in our mind. But, once we use yoga to change the negative self-talk, we see that the clients' minds and bodies may be better prepared for recovery and rehabilitation. We have seen, even 20 years after the stroke, that once the client is more accepting of who they are and where they are post-stroke, there may be space for real change in cognitive, emotional, and physical abilities.

We completed one study where clients received 16 sessions of yoga over eight weeks. An older man with stroke, named James (pseudonym), had aphasia and could follow directions and understand us but could not speak more than a few words. He mostly was able to say "Yep," and "Uh huh." James had his stroke over 20 years ago, while he was quite young. Understandably, James appeared to still be angry that he had a stroke when he was young and was frustrated with his aphasia and other disabilities. James engaged in yoga, including mantras and meditations. One day during yoga, James suddenly stated: "Arlene, shut off lights, time for yoga." This was the most complete sentence James had said in years, and it was appropriate, as I had not yet shut off the lights! James's wife broke down in tears and James looked very content, perhaps knowing he had taken steps forward in his recovery. Our team believed that it was yoga that helped James's mind and body to reconnect and to help him to be better prepared for recovery, allowing him to improve his speech, even 20 years after his stroke.

- **Dvesha: avoidance, hatred, or aversion, identification of what we don't like**. Dvesha may be considered the opposite of attachment. The ego is often involved in our hatred or aversions. Dvesha may include an avoidance of something or the development of dislike towards something; dvesha may cause distress. Anyone who has sustained a stroke does not like having had a stroke! We may feel dvesha when we are challenged, but such discomfort may also lead to growth. We must remind our clients with stroke that they will be challenged during yoga and during their recovery in general, but they cannot avoid the fact they had the stroke, nor can they avoid the fact that they will need to use yoga and other forms of rehabilitation to recover and improve.

- **Abhinivesha: fear, clinging, or attachment to life**. While all the kleshas find their foundations in avidya, they all eventually lead to and become evident as fear. For example, for clients with stroke, fear may be embedded in not fitting in, not being successful in therapy, or not fully recovering from the stroke. Regardless of where the fear is coming from or what the fear is attached to, the result is isolation and alienation from ourselves, our community, and our world.

The Eight Limbs of Yoga

There are four chapters in the Yoga Sutras and they include the eight limbs of yoga. The eight limbs of yoga are the path that Patanjali offers for a meaningful and purposeful life. In the Yoga Sutras, this pathway is called ashtanga, meaning eight limbs. Each of the limbs prepares us for the next limb or the next step, ultimately moving towards connection with the divine. While there are eight limbs of yoga, in the West, it is relatively common that only three of the eight limbs are integrated into practice (asana, pranayama, and dhyana). The eight limbs are depicted in Figure 3.1.

1. **Yamas**: Ethical standards and sense of integrity, universal practices related to "Do unto others as you would have them do unto you."

2. **Niyamas**: Self-discipline and spiritual observances, consistent yoga practice that includes meditation.

3. **Asana**: The physical postures, poses, or movements of yoga. Yoga asanas are meant to enhance discipline and the ability to concentrate. The physical practice of the asana may allow us to tap into a deep and personal energy and may be the key to enhancing post-stroke recovery. The postures create and enhance strength, balance, and flexibility.

4. **Pranayama**: Breath work to control the breath. Breath work enhances the respiratory process and connects the mind and body through connecting movement (asana) with the breath. Pranayama is the practice of controlling the breath and is often paired with movement or asanas. Prana is "life force" or "vital life force," the energy that flows through each of us. Pranayama means mastering the life force; thus, as we master our breath, we work towards mastering our life.

5. **Pratyahara**: Drawing awareness from the outside world and directing our intentions and attention internally, enhanced control of the senses.

6. **Dharana**: Concentration on a single point, enhances one's ability to concentrate and meditate.

7. **Dhyana**: The practice of meditation, being aware but without focus through a quieted mind. Providing time for meditation may mean allowing time for the integration of the practice into the body. Dhyana is the witnessing of awareness and is an important component of yoga practice.

8. **Samadhi**: Meditation to a connection with the divine. Perhaps this is the experience of joy.

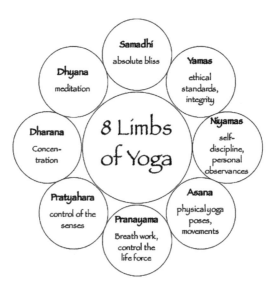

Figure 3.1

In our studies, we tend to include physical postures (asana), breath work (pranayama), meditation (dhyana), and affirmations (mantras) into the therapeutic yoga interventions we develop for clients with stroke (see Chapters 6–10 for detailed descriptions and modifications and Chapter 12 for sample yoga practices).

The Ten Yamas and Niyamas and How Each May Be Related to Stroke Recovery and Outcomes

The yamas and niyamas are found within the Yoga Sutras and are numbers one and two of the eight limbs of yoga. The yamas and niyamas may be considered a pathway to contentment and happiness, including attitudes and behaviors to guide us through our daily lives. It is thought that if one does not follow the yamas and niyamas, one will continue to suffer. Below we describe each of the yamas and niyamas, including a basic but modern definition for each and, where possible, how each yama and niyama may be associated with yoga delivered after stroke and the potential impact on recovery, outcomes, and healing.

Yamas

The yamas are ethical restraints or things to be abstained from or resisted. The yamas help us to explore and enhance our relationship with ourselves.

- **Ahimsa—non-violence, no harm**: This includes physical violence, but also the violence of words or thoughts—harmful words to ourselves or to others. We often use a lot of negative self-talk or words or thoughts telling ourselves we are not good enough or that we made so many mistakes. These thoughts may be damaging to our clients with stroke. If they are forever thinking about regrets of lifestyle or food choices that may have led to a stroke, they may never be able to fully heal or recover. Noticing our thoughts and intentions for ourselves and for others may include forgiving oneself, not being angry at the new body, or being nice to caregivers, friends, and family. Talk to clients about how to be kind to themselves in their thoughts. Once the client with stroke notices the negative thoughts, they may be able to stop feeding into the thoughts and better accept who they are. Remind clients with stroke to also be kind in their thoughts and words to others, including their caregivers and loved ones. Consider Warrior I (Virabhadrasana I) or Downward Facing Dog (Adho Mukha Svanasana) to address ahimsa (see Chapter 6).

- **Satya—truthfulness**: Being truthful, knowing that the truth is always influenced by our own experience and beliefs. Satya may also be related to integrity and acting in an honest manner at all times. In relation to stroke, perhaps satya means to be truthful or honest with oneself in regard to one's current abilities and progress after the stroke. As a yoga or rehabilitation therapist, it may also mean being truthful in regard to expectations of recovery and knowledgeable about the treatment options that are presented.

Incorporate a modified Crescent Lunge pose (Anjeneyasana) to address satya (see Chapter 6).

- **Asteya—nonstealing**: We understand that we should not take things from others or that we should not take more than we need. While we most often think of physical things, asteya also means to not steal time or happiness from others. For example, if you are late and make others wait, you are stealing time. It is important to remind ourselves and our clients to respect their own, and others', time and energy. But we are also at risk of stealing from ourselves, and perhaps this may be related to stroke recovery. In a person with stroke, perhaps asteya is related to the lack of commitment to practicing their yoga, completing their therapy, or changing to a healthier lifestyle. All of these actions would perhaps be considered stealing from possible recovery and healing, from being as whole as possible after the stroke. Consider including the mantra "I will not steal health from myself" or a modified Warrior III pose (Virabhadrasana III) if in a one-to-one therapy session and the client has strong enough balance to successfully complete the pose using a chair or a wall for balance.

- **Brahmacharya—energy moderation, continence, sustaining energy, maintenance of vitality**: The actual translation from Sanskrit to English is "celibacy," but this yama should not be associated with giving up sex. Instead, for our purposes and our time, brahmacharya may simply be to have a faithful and monogamous relationship. Relationships are often challenged after an event such as stroke, but perhaps, by doing yoga or other therapeutic practices together as a couple, relationships may be healed or enhanced. As brahmacharya may also be considered in use and moderation of energy, it is important to remind clients with stroke that fatigue is common after stroke. We should not ask our clients to use all of their energy on their yoga practice; they must become a good energy manager. Yoga asana should be used to replenish our energy storage, not deplete our energy. Child's pose (Balasana) may be used to maintain energy, facilitate relaxation, and address brahmacharya.

- **Aparigraha—non-covetousness, non-greed, nongrasping, non-attachment, non-possessiveness**: Greed may be related to material things and always wanting more. But greed may also be associated with wanting to be better than other people in a yoga class or during stroke rehabilitation. It is human nature to compare ourselves to others, but through yogic philosophy and the Yoga Sutras, we know it is better to be happy with what we have. While we want our clients with stroke to continually strive for improvements through yoga, we can also use yoga to help encourage them to be happy with their current progression, being proud and happy with their hard work and current state. Encourage the practice of not being attached to things, our practice, or improvements. Encourage being content and not overly attached to things that may be possible with yoga. Include a mantra about "I am progressing and I am happy with my progression," when using yoga as therapy to work on aparigraha.

Niyamas

The niyamas are lifestyle and active observances and were designed to create well-being for ourselves and others in our lives. The niyamas help us to grow and enhance our relationships with others.

- **Saucha—cleanliness, purity**: Keeping things clean, both inside the mind and body and outside in our surroundings. To care for the mind, using meditation (or dhyana) helps keep negative thoughts and cluttered ideas out of our minds. In our external surroundings, decreasing clutter and keeping an order to things helps us practice saucha. Additionally, decreasing clutter helps eliminate fall risks in the home after stroke. As a stroke may impact vision as well as lead to paralysis, reducing clutter in the home is a common way to manage fall risk in the home environment. One can take more care of one's body and one's space after stroke. Decreasing the clutter in our mind, body, and surroundings helps us to stop striving for perfection and may allow more time for joyful awareness. If the client is able to get to the floor and is in the chronic phase of stroke recovery, consider having them spend a few minutes in Legs Up the Wall pose (Viparita Karani) (lying in supine at a wall with the legs up the wall and the toes over the head). Also consider Downward Facing Dog (Adho Mukha Svanasana) at the wall for people with more acute stroke or who cannot easily get to the floor (see Chapter 6).

- **Santosha (sometimes samtosha)—contentment**: Being content and happy, accepting life as it currently is. It is easy in yoga to strive to always be better or do the perfect yoga pose; however, to practice santosha, we are to accept where we are in our practice and in our life. For our clients with stroke, santosha may be challenging and confusing. We are asking them to be content with their current state of having survived a stroke, but at the same time asking them to use yoga as therapy to make progress in their recovery. Santosha is to practice contentment in the moment, knowing we can move forward but being happy with our current circumstances and potentially the current post-stroke body. Bridge pose (Setu Bandha Sarvangasana) (see Chapter 6) may be included in the yoga therapy session to address santosha, perhaps with a mantra of "I am content, I am enough."

- **Tapas—self-discipline, effort, internal fire or internal heat, or spiritual austerities**: Willing to do the work and willing to learn. The heat that the work and the learning create burns away impurities while simultaneously sparking the divinity within. Committing to the work of a yoga practice, or other post-stroke therapy, and really doing it every day as planned, is tapas. Committing to healthy habits, such as a healthy diet or routinely taking important blood pressure medicine, may be important tapas after stroke. Tapas is also related to finding and knowing one's own determination and will (will power), important when asking a person with post-stroke disability to engage in yoga as therapy. Tapas is inner heat, which is thought to cleanse the body; asanas that create heat will help to address tapas during the therapy sessions for people with stroke.

- **Svadhyaya—a self-study exploring one's own person, mind, body, and spirit**: A purposeful and meaningful study of self to find the happiness that lies within each of us. Really looking in and studying ourselves helps us to better understand our patterns of doing and feeling. It is common for people who have sustained a stroke to turn inward and perhaps consider why they had a stroke and why they survived a stroke, but they may not look inward to find their happiness or what they may be grateful for. Svadhyaya helps us to each better understand complex life experiences and increase compassion for others but also for ourselves. Self-compassion is of great importance to people who have sustained a stroke and who are working hard in their recovery and healing. If possible, help the client to move into Easy pose (Sukhasana) (see Chapter 6) to allow space for svadhyaya or self-study.

- **Ishvara pranidhana—dedicate, surrender, or devotion to a higher power**: The highest happiness. Ishvara pranidhana may be considered the big picture or ultimate goal of yoga. Importantly, ishvara pranidhana helps us to receive the grace of simply being alive. Additionally, this niyama helps us to shift our thoughts away from "I" and "me" and helps to settle the mind. A person after stroke may feel great frustration and many agitations of the mind related to the stroke and their recovery. Yoga may help them focus less on the "I had a stroke," or "I can't do something because of my stroke," and more on "I am alive after a stroke," or "I am recovering from my stroke," allowing for a shift in their "stroke story" and allowing them to move on to recovery. Prayer pose (Anjali Mudra), or hands at Namaste, represents ishvara pranidhana and is likely included in all yoga sessions.

If readers would like a fun way to learn the yamas and niyamas, check out the yama and niyama song on YouTube by Tom Gillette.

The Koshas

We, as humans, are complex and have many layers to us. In yogic philosophy, these layers are often compared to sheaths or the layers of an onion and are called the koshas (see Figure 3.2). There are five koshas to consider in yoga and they address the physical to the spiritual being. By understanding the koshas, the yoga or rehabilitation therapist can best deliver yoga as a holistic treatment, addressing the whole person. Where possible, we link the koshas to the use of yoga for therapy after stroke.

- **Annamaya kosha**: The "foodstuff" or "physical matter" sheath or body. "Maya" translates to "made of." This kosha is most often addressed through asanas or physical yoga postures. This is the kosha of the physical self and is nourished by food and physical activity. A healthy diet helps to keep the body nourished but may also help with recovery after stroke. Importantly, a healthy diet will also help with the prevention of a future stroke. Stroke prevention is related to management of both blood pressure and diabetes; both are associated with diet. Taking care of the physical body, using the physical postures of yoga as a physical activity, also helps to improve and maintain the physical self after a stroke. In our own research (Schmid, *et al.*, 2014), we have found that the physical postures of yoga, or asanas, are known to improve many levels of physical functioning, including balance, strength, range of motion, pain, gait speed, and walking endurance. It is also known that yoga improves other aspects of physical functioning, including digestion and elimination, heart and lung function, and other physical systems of the body.

- **Pranamaya kosha**: The "energy" sheath or body. Prana is the "life force," the "vital force," or the "life energy" and is commonly referred to during yoga. This kosha is most often addressed through breath work. Our breath is the "life force" within us and is vital to recovery and wellness. The prana, or the "life force," is what connects the mind and the body. Connecting the breath with movement is paramount in any yoga practice but is particularly necessary when working with clients with stroke. The mind-body disconnect that seems to occur after stroke may be minimized with yoga that includes asana and breath work, particularly Alternate Nostril Breathing (Nadi Shodhana Pranayama).

- **Manomaya kosha**: The "mind-stuff" sheath or mental/emotional body. This kosha includes the mind and five sensory organs and makes up the "personhood." The manomaya kosha allows for the diversity in each of us and our emotional ups and downs. There are many emotions that may occur after stroke; many clients with stroke and their caregivers may express gratefulness for being alive. However, depression and anxiety may develop and may be due to changes in the brain or may be related to the stroke and potential losses or changes that may occur or changes that have already occurred for people with chronic stroke. This kosha is most often addressed through deep relaxation and meditation. Using meditation, breath for relaxation, and other yoga practices to be more in the present moment and more content helps to improve anxiety and depression after a stroke.

- **Vijnanamaya kosha:** The "wisdom" sheath or the knowledge body. The vijnanamaya kosha is our intellect or the higher mind and is associated with perception. It is important for the yoga or rehabilitation therapist to remember that knowledge and intellect are fluid, especially after a stroke. Working with clients so that they keep an open mind and are ready to try new things will help them navigate through the world with their new post-stroke mind and body. Cognitive changes are common after stroke, and clients, and their families, may be frustrated with changes in their mental capacities.

- **Anandamaya kosha:** The "bliss" sheath or body. To address our bliss sheath, know that we as humans must find contentment. Often after stroke, people are not content with their new mind and body. Yoga may help bring contentment and move individuals closer to finding bliss. Remind clients and their family members to find bliss or happiness in their everyday lives; remind them to be grateful for just how far they have come in their recovery.

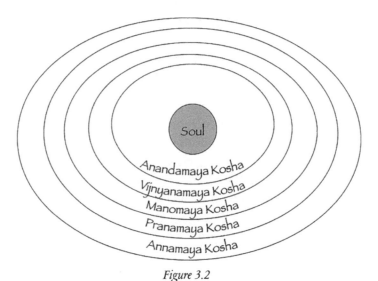

Figure 3.2

While the koshas are described as layers, they do not really operate in this manner or as independent entities. Rather, they are interdependent and work together to form the whole person. Therefore, it is important to use yoga to address all five of the koshas and acknowledge that change may happen throughout any or all of the koshas.

The Chakras

The chakras are energy centers recognized in our bodies, which essentially are channels for energy flow. While most yogic traditions identify seven chakras, Kundalini yoga identifies eight (described below). The chakras are said to interact with the physiologic and neurologic systems of the body and the chakras help to regulate the complex processes that occur in the body. Each chakra is depicted with a color and an icon or picture and they run from the crown of the head to the base of the spine. Yoga may be used to help balance the chakras or to keep the chakras healthy and allow energy to flow through each.

For each of the chakras we include both yoga postures and mantras that may be used to balance the chakra. We identify a few yoga postures for each chakra that are appropriate and/or modifiable for most clients with stroke. Some of the included postures are more challenging and may not be suitable for a group setting but require one-to-one teaching or therapy to maintain safety and decrease the risk of injury. See Chapters 6 and 7 for more information on each of the identified poses. We include one or two mantras to work on for each of the chakras as well. See Figure 3.3 to further examine the seven traditional chakras.

- **Root chakra**: The root chakra is also known as muladhara. Our root chakra is at the base of the spine in the tailbone area and it represents our ability to feel grounded, our foundation, or our connection to the earth. The root chakra is associated with survival issues such as food and money. It is likely that the root chakra is impacted after stroke, secondary to the changes in communication between the brain and the body. Changes to the physical body, including challenged balance, strength, flexibility, and mobility, may disrupt the root chakra. By working with the root chakra, we are able to ground the body and connect to our sense of security, stability, and safety. This grounding may have a positive impact on mobility but also on the feeling of security and safety, allowing for less fear of falling or less fear of a future stroke. Standing postures, including balance poses, along with Bridge pose (Setu Bandha Sarvangasana) and Knees to Chest pose (Apanasana) (see Chapter 6), provide help with grounding and are used to balance the root chakra. A mantra may include "I am safe," or "I am strong and I am stable." The root chakra is often represented by the color red.

- **Sacral chakra**: The sacral chakra, or svadhishthana, is our connection and ability to accept others and new experiences. It is located in the lower abdomen, about two inches below the navel and two inches into the body. The sacral chakra is associated with emotional issues such as a sense of abundance, well-being, pleasure, and sexuality. Working with the sacral chakras helps us to create a balance or connection between the body and the mind. Cobra pose (Bhujangasana), Chair pose (Utkatasana), Locust pose (Salabhasana), or Forward Folds (Paschimottanasana) (see Chapter 6) may be helpful in working with the sacral chakra. A mantra for the sacral chakra may include "I am well and I have enough," or "I am creative." The sacral chakra is represented by the color orange.

- **Solar plexus chakra**: The solar plexus chakra, also known as manipura, is located in the upper abdomen area, between the navel and the lower end of the sternum. This chakra represents our ability to be confident and in control of our own lives. The solar plexus chakra is related to our self-worth, self-confidence, and self-esteem. Working with the solar plexus chakra may help to encourage positive and empowered thinking, important for our clients after a stroke. Modified Boat (Navasana), Cat Cow (Chakravakasana), Warrior I and II (Virabhadrasana I and II), and twisting postures (see Chapter 6) may be useful poses in working with the solar plexus chakra. The mantra "I am enough" may be used to work with the solar plexus chakra. The color yellow represents the solar plexus chakra.

- **Heart chakra**: The heart chakra represents our ability to love and is found at the center of the chest, just above the heart. The heart chakra is also called the anahata. The heart chakra is also connected to the lungs and the thymus gland. The heart chakra is associated with love, joy, and inner peace. Working with this chakra may help to balance our nervous system and help our minds to focus, important issues to address after a stroke. Cat Cow (Chakravakasana), Eagle (Garudasana), or Upward Facing Dog (Urdha Mukha Svanasana) poses (see Chapter 6) may be used when working to balance the heart chakra. Mantras to include while working on the heart chakra may include "I am loved," or "I have compassion for myself and for others." The heart chakra is green in color and is thought to be the most balancing of the chakras.

- **Throat chakra**: The throat chakra is our ability to communicate and is located in the throat. Vishuddha is the Sanskrit name for the throat chakra. Because the throat chakra acts as a channel between the heart and the mind, this chakra is linked to our communication and our self-expression of feelings. Neck flexion, extension, lateral flexion, and rotation may be used in balancing the throat chakra. Bridge pose (Setu Bandha Sarvangasana) and Child's pose (Balasana) (see Chapter 6) may also be helpful when working on the throat chakra. The addition of mantras spoken out loud may also be helpful in working with the throat chakra. Mantras to include may be "I am heard," or "I express myself." The color blue represents the throat chakra.

- **Third eye chakra**: The third eye chakra, or ajna, is located in the forehead between the eyes (between the eyebrows) and allows us the ability to focus on and see the big picture. The third eye chakra is the seat for intuition and wisdom but is also associated with the pituitary gland, which is linked to our sleeping cycles. Emotional issues related to the third eye chakra include intuition, imagination, wisdom, and, importantly, our abilities to think and to make decisions. Poses to work on the third eye chakra after stroke may include Downward Facing Dog (Adho Mukha Svanasana), Child's pose (Balasana), or Standing Half Forward Fold (Ardha Uttanasana). Alternate Nostril Breathing (Nadi Shodhana Pranayama) is also used to work with the third eye chakra. Mantras to include may be "My mind is calm," or "My mind is open to new ideas." The third eye chakra is represented by the color indigo.

- **Crown chakra**: The crown chakra is located at the very top, or crown, of our head and is related to the pineal gland in the brain. The crown chakra is also named the sahasrara and may be considered our own spiritual connection. This chakra bridges the two hemispheres of the brain. After a stroke, we frequently want to help the client activate both brain hemispheres, and perhaps working with the crown chakra is a way to do so. The crown chakra is associated with our inner and outer beauty and our spiritual connection. Many of the yoga poses used to address the crown chakra are inversions (think headstand or plow) and are likely not appropriate after a stroke. The Seated Forward Fold (Upavistha Konasana) is, however, a yoga pose that benefits the crown chakra while still being a safe pose. A mantra to include may be "I surrender to what I do not know or do not understand." The color violet represents the crown chakra.

- **Aura**: In the Kundalini yoga tradition, the eighth chakra is the aura. An aura is the electromagnetic field, or the energy field, of all beings. The aura is associated with health, and all organs and elements impact the aura. The color of the aura changes based on emotional, physical, and mental states. The human challenge and gift of the aura is to experience "one's energetic self" and the sole desire is to identify with the soul. All meditations are thought to enhance the aura, as is Downward Facing Dog (Adho Mukha Svanasana) (called triangle in Kundalini yoga), all arm exercises, and Kundalini postures of archer and ego eradicator. Mantras to target the aura may include "I am strong, I am healthy, I am vibrant."

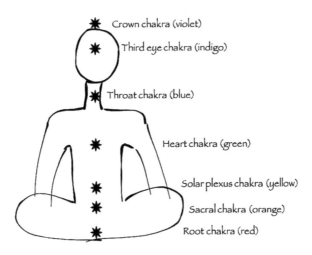

Figure 3.3

In summary, the chakras are all associated with important properties. In stroke recovery and rehabilitation, we may be able to address certain issues by focusing the yoga practice or mantras on certain chakras.

The Vayus

There are five movements or functions of prana (life force), called the vayus. Vayu is translated to mean "wind" or "direction of energy," and each vayu moves energy, or prana, through our bodies in a specific direction. In yogic philosophies, prana is what allows us to move our bodies and to think with our minds. But prana also allows us to coordinate our senses and energy, allowing our nervous and organ systems to work together and to function. The five vayus maintain and repair different areas of the body and the necessary functions of our bodies. In essence, the vayus govern or regulate different aspects of our bodies. As in previous sections, we include yoga postures for each of the vayus that we identify as appropriate and/or modifiable for most clients with stroke. Some of the postures may not be suitable for a group setting as they are more challenging. As appropriate, the more challenging poses should be delivered in one-to-one therapy sessions. See Chapter 6 for more information on each of the identified poses.

- **Prana vayu:** The prana vayu moves energy all around, governs inhalation, and is the fundamental energy in the body. Prana vayu also governs the intake of all things, including food, air, senses, and thoughts. Anxiety and fear are present when prana vayu is not balanced. This vayu is centered in the chest and the head, and the energy nourishes the brain and the eyes. Connecting breath to movement and reminding clients to not hold their breath during challenging poses is a way to support prana vayu while using yoga poses for clients after stroke. Consider including Warrior I (Virabhadrasana I), Chair pose (Utkatasana), or back bends/back extension to balance the prana vayu.

- **Samana vayu:** The samana vayu moves energy inward and governs the digestive system, focusing digestion, absorption, and assimilation of food, drink, air, and experiences that come into the body. The samana vayu is in the abdomen, centered in the navel. When samana is not balanced or is blocked, clients may have difficulties thinking about or talking about challenging experiences, for example the time of the stroke or the post-stroke recovery. Seated Forward Folds (Upavistha Konasana) and Spinal Twist (Jathara Parivartanasana) may be used to address the samana vayu.

- **Apana vayu:** The apana vayu moves energy downward and is centered in the lower abdominal region and the pelvis. Apana vayu governs elimination from the body (urine, carbon monoxide, etc.) and downward and outward movement. It is experienced when we are grounded. Energy from the apana vayu nourishes the digestion, reproduction, and elimination organs. Standing poses, Seated Forward Folds (Upavistha Konasana), and seated twists are all poses to work with the apana vayu, ultimately enhancing elimination.

- **Udana vayu:** The udana vayu moves energy upward. The udana vayu is centered in the diaphragm and moves prana upward through the lungs, bronchi, and the throat. This vayu governs exhalation and is expressed through growth, communication, expansion, expression, and ascension. Udana vayu helps us to move our emotions, including negative emotions, up and out of ourselves. Yoga poses that allow the client to experience vayu are Staff pose (Rekha) or Chair pose (Utkatasana).

- **Vyana vayu:** The vyana vayu moves energy outward and is the core of the body, near the heart. Energy from vyana flows through the entire body. It is the opposite of samana vayu. This vayu governs circulation on all levels, moving energy in and out of the extremities, and works with the blood, lymphatic, and nervous systems. This vayu includes some regulation of emotions. Postures to use with the client to balance the vyana vayu include lateral side bending and Corpse pose (Savasana).

Summary

Yoga has the power to treat the whole person. Yoga is much more than just the physical postures, and to be most effectively used as therapy after a stroke, it must also include breath work, meditation, and affirmations (mantras). We suggest that rehabilitation therapists who want to use yoga in their practice learn about yogic philosophies to be better grounded in using yoga as therapy or to consider becoming a yoga teacher or yoga therapist. The next chapter further explores the research that has been completed in regard to yoga for clients with stroke.

CHAPTER 4

Evidence-Based Research Supporting the Use of Yoga as Therapy After Stroke

Research 101 for Yoga After Stroke

A fair amount of research has been completed regarding the benefits of yoga for people who have sustained a stroke. Of great importance, researchers have found that yoga is feasible for people with stroke, and that people with stroke can in fact successfully complete a yoga practice. This means that, in our research, we have found that clients with stroke, even a stroke that is decades old, can complete yoga physical postures (including mudras and eye movements), can engage in breath work, are able to repeat mantras, and are able to finish the yoga session in Corpse pose (Savasana), relax, and meditate. Often, clients with stroke need help with postures, modifications, or props, or assistance to get to and from the floor, but they can do it! They can also complete yoga without standing up or getting to the floor, doing the entire yoga session in bed or in a chair. Yoga is very adaptable, and we can accommodate the needs of the individual client with stroke; see Figure 4.1.

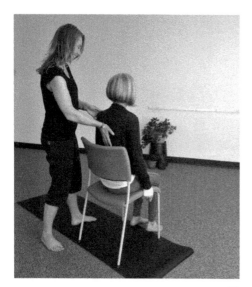 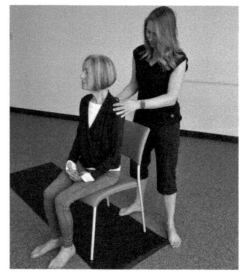

Figure 4.1

In general, the research that has been completed supports the use of yoga as an intervention for clients with stroke. The research evidence supports that yoga improves cognitive, emotional, and physical well-being after stroke and, importantly, also improves functional outcomes and quality of life. Therefore, we encourage the use of yoga postures, breath work, mantras, and meditation as an evidence-based practice after stroke. For example, in our research we observed changes in multiple outcomes. Often there are statistically significant improvements in measured objective outcomes with just two classes each week for eight weeks of yoga (16 sessions in total). Importantly, not all are measured quantitative outcomes, but clients often self-report subjective changes that have occurred throughout the yoga intervention. We have seen improvements in cognitive, emotional, and physical changes that commonly occur after a stroke, including:

- cognitive changes:
  - improved processing time
  - more concrete thinking and memory
  - improved ability to attend to conversation or tasks
  - improved perception
  - better motor planning or ability to follow instructions
  - enhanced social cognitive or emotional intelligence
  - decision-making abilities
  - communication, including reading, speaking, and understanding speech
  - seeing or understanding what someone is seeing
  - fewer perceived constraints to engaging in activities or trying new activities
- emotional changes:
  - feeling less frustrated
  - feeling less anxious
  - feeling less depressed
  - more stable mood or improved emotional regulation
  - less likely to cry, or crying for more appropriate reasons
  - ability to be less reactive or have a more appropriate response to an event
  - feeling more like the old self
  - improved confidence or self-efficacy

- physical changes:

  - improved sensations, including decreased paralysis and enhanced proprioception

  - improvements in motor control

  - less asymmetry

  - less fatigue

  - improved vision, including the ability to see and read

  - decreased pain

  - improved balance and balance confidence

  - improved balance

  - decreased fall risks, being more mindful about listening to their body and where their body is in space

  - improved gait speed and endurance

  - improved upper and lower body flexibility

  - improved upper and lower body strength

  - improved range of motion.

Perhaps most important are the recorded improvements we see in overall function, including activities of daily living and quality of life. Clients also make statements that indicate an enhanced mind-body connection; however, they do not necessarily use these words. Other clients talk about being more mindful in their everyday lives or about using a calming pranayama when they are stressed about something in life. It seems that for many clients in our studies, yoga has become an integral aspect of their day-to-day lives.

A Bit of Caution

We are therapists and researchers, but we are not medical doctors. Our experience with yoga is both from our personal use of yoga and using yoga in our research and our clinical practice. If there is concern or worry about a person with stroke beginning to use yoga, we believe the therapist should help them reach out to their physician to make sure that yogic practices are approved and not contraindicated. It is ultimately up to the therapist and the client to determine if and when yoga is an appropriate treatment option after stroke.

The Research

While we embed research evidence throughout this book in order to help the yoga or rehabilitation therapist use evidence-based yoga interventions where possible, here we provide a simple synopsis of the literature published through 2017. There are many studies that influence the stroke rehabilitation literature or the older adult literature, but there are only approximately ten published articles that focus on yoga as an intervention for clients with stroke; we review each here. Much of the yoga literature is under-developed and includes small sample sizes or lacks control groups; this is simply because, while yoga is 5000 years old, yoga and yoga as therapy are relatively new topics of research.

Yoga for Other Populations

As there is limited research specific to yoga and stroke, we include a review of some other yoga literature, including yoga for older adults, yoga in the inpatient rehabilitation setting, and yoga for brain injury (as stroke is a type of brain injury).

Yoga and Older Adults

Due to the large amount of studies completed in regard to adults and older adults, here we discuss published systematic reviews of the literature (or even reviews of the systematic reviews). A systematic review means that authors have reviewed and synthesized all published research that addresses the efficacy or effectiveness of an intervention. In 2013, McCall, *et al.* published a review of systematic reviews regarding the use of yoga for adults with acute and chronic health conditions. The authors stated that they reviewed 26 systematic reviews and that, while overall the quality of the evidence was low, there was developing evidence for the use of yoga as a therapeutic intervention. The review identified that yoga may be quite effective in reducing symptoms of anxiety, depression, and pain. Unfortunately, stroke was not included as one of the chronic health conditions in the review. Desveaux, *et al.* (2015) completed a separate review of the yoga literature pertinent to the use of yoga to manage chronic disease. The authors included a meta-analysis of ten yoga intervention studies and did include stroke as a diagnosis. The authors focused the review on exercise capacity, health-related quality of life, anxiety, and depression. Across diagnostic populations (stroke, heart disease, and chronic obstructive pulmonary disorder), the authors concluded that yoga had a positive effect on both exercise capacity and health-related quality of life. However, specifically in the studies that were focused on stroke, likely due to the high variability among stroke studies and outcome measures, the authors of the meta-analysis could not determine the impact of yoga on exercise capacity or depression after stroke. The authors indicated that yoga led to improvements in post-stroke health-related quality of life and anxiety. The authors also concluded that yoga may be a helpful addition to rehabilitation.

Patel, Newstead, and Ferrer (2012) published a systematic review and meta-analysis of yoga interventions for older adults, specifically addressing the impact of yoga on health-related quality of life and physical functioning. The review included 18 studies that included adults over the age of 60 years old. The dose of yoga varied as well as the characteristics and co-morbidities of the study populations. The authors concluded that yoga may be superior to other more conventional physical activity interventions for older adults. We tested yoga as an intervention in older adults and found improvements in dynamic balance and reductions in fear of falling (Schmid, et al., 2010; Van Puymbroeck, et al., 2017).

Yoga During Inpatient Rehabilitation

We also completed a qualitative study where we integrated yoga therapy into ongoing inpatient rehabilitation (Schmid, et al., 2015b; Van Puymbroeck, et al., 2015). We recruited 53 individuals in just three months from two local rehabilitation facilities. Both rehabilitation facilities treated clients with acute injuries or medical events. In the study, we included any patient who wished to be included, regardless of diagnosis, but this did include individuals with acute stroke. Even though many of the study participants had substantial physical limitations, they were each able to engage in modified yoga postures and/or breath work. Study participants overwhelmingly indicated improvement in breath control, body responsiveness, and being able to better focus on their recovery and therapy; 97% of all study participants recommended yoga therapy to other individuals with disabilities. Additionally, we interviewed the rehabilitation therapists and key administration personnel to examine their perceptions of the feasibility and the utility of integrating yoga into inpatient rehabilitation (Van Puymbroeck, et al., 2015). Issues around policy and organizational considerations were apparent, and some key personnel did not feel well informed about the project. Importantly though, in general, therapists and administration personnel thought that integrating yoga into inpatient rehabilitation was feasible and beneficial to clients receiving care in an inpatient rehabilitation center. Rehabilitation therapists in particular discussed the benefits of yoga being a holistic approach and a way to treat the whole person after a significant life event, such as a stroke. One therapist stated:

> I really liked the, like I had mentioned, the holistic approach that that had brought on. So, bringing that aspect where, um, we don't always have time to, um, utilize that in our intervention or even just to be able to, uh, teach them some of those basic breathing and relaxation techniques. Um, I just thought that was a great adjunct to that program as a whole. (Van Puymbroeck, et al., 2015, p.3)

One therapist talked about how yoga helped to reduce stress for some clients and that the clients learned to calm themselves down during stressful times or painful treatments. The therapist said:

> Most of my patients…I referred for relaxation and those things and they kind of seemed to benefit from that. Especially breathing techniques; they were all very pleased with those things. Just learning you know, about how to focus on breathing,

how to calm themselves down and maintain stress and anxiety. So, those things are the things that seemed to help. (Van Puymbroeck, *et al.*, 2015, p.4)

Additionally, a therapist talked about how yoga could be used to improve camaraderie among patients, allowing them to get to know each other in a group setting. The therapist stated:

I mean the individual [session] is important but I think I could see it more as an adjunct to doing groups. You know, because we don't do those things anymore. We used to have a lot of groups. It was a good source of camaraderie and getting to know other people. (Van Puymbroeck, *et al.*, 2015, p.3)

Yoga After Brain Injury

As stroke is a type of brain injury, we provide a brief review of the literature related to yoga interventions for clients with brain injuries. We completed a case study of yoga for people with chronic traumatic brain injury. Yoga was delivered by a yoga therapist and provided in a one-to-one format for 16 sessions. While quantitative and qualitative data from our study support the occurrence of multiple improvements, most notable were the improvements in balance. After eight weeks of yoga, each of the three individuals participating in the study demonstrated improved balance. As a group, there was a 36% improvement in balance scores (Schmid, *et al.*, 2016a). We also saw improvements in emotional regulation and health-related quality of life (Grimm, *et al.*, 2017). We recently completed a study to assess whether yoga could be delivered to clients with brain injury in a group format. Our results indicate that the study participants enjoyed being with each other and learning from each other, that group yoga was feasible, and that participants showed improvements in physical and emotional outcomes, as well as quality of life (Roney, *et al.*, under review).

Other researchers have also studied yoga after brain injury, but these studies are also small and typically without control groups (Donnelly, *et al.*, 2017; Silverthorne, *et al.*, 2012). In 2015, Gerber and Gargaro had clients with brain injury participate in activities, including the option for yoga, over a six-month period. Study participants showed increased community integration and their families experienced a decrease in family burden of care. In a pilot study of the effects of breath-focused yoga for adults with severe traumatic brain injury, participants self-reported improvements in physical functioning, emotional well-being, and overall health over time. Their results further substantiate the value of yoga for individuals with traumatic brain injury. In a different pilot study, researchers explored adapted yoga and found significant improvements in the Emotions and Feelings subscales of the Quality-of-Life After Brain Injury instrument among individuals with acquired brain injury who participated in yoga compared with individuals who did not receive yoga. The control group participants did not significantly improve in the same outcome measures. These improvements indicated increased emotional satisfaction and decreased negative emotions after participating in the yoga intervention.

Meditation and the Brain

Meditation, a key component of yoga, has been frequently studied and has been found to manage multiple symptoms, but most often these are emotional symptoms. Meditation and mindful meditation have yet to be studied in clients without stroke, except when meditation is included as part of yoga. Interestingly, however, there is exciting scientific evidence proving neural changes in normal adults after meditation; for example, neuroimaging has been shown to improve connectivity in the brain and increase cortical thickness, as well as increase actual size or thickness in brain gray matter (Hölzel, *et al.*, 2011; Lazar, *et al.*, 2000, 2005). Moss and colleagues (2012) completed a study in people with mild cognitive impairment and included eight weeks of yoga and a Kirtan Kriya meditation. The meditation included mudras and chanting the "Sa Ta Na Ma" meditation. The meditation was 12 minutes long and was to be completed daily. While the sample was small and included 15 people in the study, results showed improvements in mood, anxiety, tension, and fatigue. Importantly, these changes were correlated with changes in the blood flow in the brain. It is essential to pull evidence larger than just yoga and stroke literature, as there are so few studies specific to a yoga intervention for only people with stroke.

Yoga After Stroke

The stroke literature indicates that recovery is possible during the chronic stages of stroke due to neuroplasticity. It is, however, necessary that clients with chronic stroke have the opportunity to engage in novel or new exercise programming to allow for further recovery (Page, Gater, and Bach-y-Rita, 2004). Yoga is a novel exercise intervention that treats the whole person and has the potential to be highly effective at improving multiple outcome measures for people with stroke.

Two case studies specific to yoga and stroke have been published. One study included four people with stroke, and the other had three clients with stroke (Bastille and Gill-Body, 2004; Lynton, Kligler, and Shiflett, 2007). Case studies are a necessary first step of research, documenting that an intervention such as yoga is feasible with a new or complex patient population, such as clients with stroke. Bastille and Gill-Body included four participants, each with chronic stroke and hemiparesis. Clients each completed bi-weekly yoga sessions for eight weeks and demonstrated improved balance (clinically significant on the Berg Balance Scale), timed movements (Timed Movement Battery), and scoring on the following Stroke Impact Scale domains: physical; cognitive; emotional; and social participation. The second case study, completed by Lynton, *et al.*, included three people with stroke. Each client received 12 weeks of yoga. Each of the three subjects improved in dexterity (the O'Connor Tweezer Dexterity Test) and speech (Boston Diagnostic Aphasia Exam) scores. The results of the case studies paved the way for the future of yoga intervention research.

Garrett, Immink, and Hillier (2011) completed a qualitative study to look at the lived experience of clients with stroke who each completed a yoga intervention.

Results from the qualitative analyses indicated that the clients perceived improvements in strength, range of motion, and their gait. Perhaps more importantly, clients discussed the acceptance of their post-stroke "different body" and that the yoga helped to reconnect the mind and body after the stroke. Garrett, *et al.* is the first group to discuss the mind-body connection in clients with stroke. The complex systems of the brain and body require integration of the mind and multiple body functions, structures, and systems to work most effectively (Weerdesteyn, *et al.*, 2008). It therefore stands to reason that yoga, which involves a holistic mind-body intervention, is capable of simultaneously targeting multiple systems and would be a most effective intervention after stroke.

Much of our yoga intervention research has focused on improving balance, strength, and range of motion in the lower extremities in order to decrease post-stroke fall rates. To date, our study was the largest yoga trial completed for clients with stroke, was published in a high impact journal (*Stroke*), and received extensive media attention. It is, however, important to note that while our study included a control group, the participants in that group only received usual care. This means the participants in the control group did not receive any additional training or intervention but continued as "usual" or normal with their healthcare trajectory. Study participants randomized to the usual care control group were then offered eight weeks of yoga after the control period was completed. Future studies with stronger control groups are necessary, but our research demonstrated that yoga was both feasible and beneficial to clients with chronic stroke (Schmid, *et al.*, 2012, 2014).

Due to significant fall rates and unaddressed fall risk factors after a stroke, our study aims were to improve balance and fall risk factors, such as confidence, strength, and range of motion. There is an established relationship between balance and hip and ankle range of motion in older adults and in people with stroke (Chiacchiero, *et al.*, 2010; Kerrigan, *et al.*, 1998, 2001). By developing yoga programming to directly influence lower extremity balance, strength, and range of motion, we were able to show that yoga improves balance confidence (confidence to maintain balance) and addresses other fall risk factors (Schmid, *et al.*, 2012, 2014). Learn about the benefits of different yoga poses by reviewing Hand Out 13.3. We developed the yoga intervention with the help of Nancy Schalk, a yoga therapist in Indianapolis, IN, who has years of experience practicing with people with disabilities. We chose each pose and the flow of the poses based on stroke rehabilitation research, as well as the benefits of each yoga posture and breath. In the development of the eight-week yoga intervention, we had to consider the best postures and breath work to include to best meet our aims, but we also had to consider postures that were most likely to be feasible for people with chronic stroke to complete. See the sample practices in Chapter 12 for the identified yoga poses, breath work, meditation, and mantras that we included in this research study.

Balance, and other outcome measures, significantly improved for the clients randomized to the eight-week yoga intervention. Additionally, there was even a meaningful clinical difference in balance scores, meaning that the change in balance decreased clients' risk of falling. However, we know that yoga is so much more than only improving the physical body. In this randomized controlled pilot study that included the usual care control group, for clients randomized to the yoga intervention, we found improvements in upper and lower strength and range of motion, endurance, balance, balance confidence, and pain, but we also found improvements in quality of life (Schmid, *et al.*, 2012, 2014). We also found that clients with better attendance (more yoga) had better outcomes in some measures, including balance confidence.

In the same randomized trial of yoga after stroke, we also assessed the impact of yoga on postural stability (Altenburger, *et al.*, 2016; Miller, *et al.*, 2015). In these analyses, 21 of the study participants completed electronic assessments of their balance. We found improvement in weight distribution, meaning the clients were more equally distributing their weight into both legs, including the leg with hemiparesis. Additionally, clients in the study who completed yoga showed more than a 50% improvement in symmetrical alignment in their lower extremities during different standing positions. Changes in weight distribution and asymmetries have been linked to balance and fall rates after a stroke, and these changes may be why the clients in the study demonstrated such improvements in balance.

Just as important as the quantitative data and physical performance measures was the qualitative data we collected to hear about the experience of being in a yoga intervention study after a stroke. Clients randomized to the yoga intervention talked about how yoga improved their day-to-day life and that as their balance, strength, and range of motion improved, they began to go back out into their world and communities. Some clients talked about being able to go out with friends and family again. A man who had very impaired mobility found that he could walk to the park, and he was able to walk to the bus stop and get on the bus. Once he could get on the bus, his entire community was once again open to him. One man was even able to climb the stairs in his house for the first time since his stroke, and he was able to once again sleep in the same bed as his wife. Other study participants talked about how they felt more like themselves than at any time since before the stroke. Still others told us about how they no longer cried uncontrollably. Other study participants talked about how yoga concurrently allowed them to improve and to be content with where they were in their lives and their yoga practice. Still others found that yoga improved their ability to see or to read. We have not captured all of these outcomes with hard objective data, but the subjective qualitative data tells us that eight weeks of yoga truly changed lives (Van Puymbroeck, *et al.*, 2014)! In Table 4.1 we provide numerous quotes about both the satisfaction with the yoga intervention and the improvements that occurred after the intervention.

Table 4.1: Selected qualitative supportive comments from our study of yoga for participants with stroke

Feasibility, acceptability, and satisfaction of the yoga intervention
• "You got to be balanced. And know how far you can go. This couldn't have been any better."
• "This was great, it was important to the whole therapy process… It should definitely be added to other therapies."
• "Now I tell everyone they should do yoga, it has helped everything."
• "After therapy…basically send you out the door…something like this should be mandatory. There I felt like half a person. Here I feel like 90–95% of a person. I'd like to see the program extended."
• "It's probably one of the best things that [has] ever come to me."
• "That's the best part about this program; no pain. You don't do anything that's painful. And you still get better."

Improved balance, QoL, and related outcomes
• "I remember first getting home from the hospital… I would get so anxious and so nervous about stuff you know…thinking, how am I going to do that? I think with this program that doesn't even enter into it anymore."
• "I've gone upstairs in my house about three times in the past week, and I hadn't been upstairs in a couple months. I have a real fear of stairs, and this gave me more confidence in balance and holding on."
• "I'm able to walk down the stairs, used to slither down… It's given me confidence."
• "I'm gonna cry…it's improved my life, I can take a shower, before I couldn't. I was scared."
• "I am still doing yoga, and now I am going walking, I never would have thought I could do anything after my stroke. This gave me the courage to be active, to exercise."

Authors of a more recently published randomized controlled trial recruited 22 clients with a chronic stroke (at least nine months after the occurrence of the stroke). Study participants were randomized into a ten-week yoga intervention group or a usual care control group (Immink, Hillier, and Petkov, 2014). The ten-week yoga intervention included weekly 90-minute sessions. The yoga program was developed for clients with stroke and the chosen postures and breath work focused on promoting a light-intensity activity, sensory and movement awareness, relaxation, and enhancement of a positive mood. The developed yoga intervention included yoga postures, breath work practices, and meditation, and postures were modified as needed. A home practice was included and encouraged. There were no differences between groups, which is likely due to the small sample size. Clients randomized to the yoga intervention group did benefit from significant improvements in quality of life (assessed with the Stroke Impact Scale) and perceived motor functional recovery. Motor function recovery was assessed with the 9-Hole Peg Test, the Motor Assessment Scale, Berg Balance Scale, 2-Minute Walk Test, and the Comfortable Gait Speed Test. While not statistically significant, there were clinically relevant changes in anxiety (anxiety was measured with the State Trait Anxiety Inventory).

Other researchers have focused on the impact of yoga on post-stroke depression and anxiety (Chan, Immink, and Hillier, 2012). The researchers included 14 individuals with chronic stroke and randomized study participants to receive exercise or exercise plus yoga. Individuals randomized to yoga received weekly yoga classes for six weeks with a yoga home exercise program included. All study participants also were invited to a group exercise class, also for six weeks. The sample was not large enough to determine statistically significant differences between the two groups, but clients in the yoga plus exercise group had greater improvements in anxiety and depression than the exercise-only group. Of course, clients who received yoga plus exercise had more prescribed active time, had more time out of their homes spent with other people with stroke, and had more access to the group leader. The impact of yoga on anxiety and depression cannot be fully determined, but these constructs may be further studied in future yoga research studies.

We have included Alternate Nostril Breathing in all of our yoga studies. Nadi Shodhana Pranayama is the Sanskrit name for Alternate Nostril Breathing and means "subtle energy clearing breathing technique." Researchers studied the use of Alternate Nostril Breathing in 11 clients with stroke (Marshall, *et al.*, 2014), as this breathing technique has, in neuro-typical adults, led to improved verbal and spatial cognition. Of the 11 study participants, approximately half had some level of diagnosable aphasia. All study participants received training in Alternate Nostril Breathing for four weeks and were then asked to continue the practice on their own for the next six weeks. Study participants were asked to use Alternate Nostril Breathing at least six days a week and attempted to progress to 40-minute sessions. There was a significant decrease in anxiety after the yoga intervention, and those study participants who had aphasia also demonstrated improved communication and language abilities. We have not measured communication or aspects of aphasia in our studies. However, we hear time and again that many of our study participants perceive improvements in communication abilities—for example, they have qualitatively reported: improved number of words they can say; increased ability to string more words together; and better processing of information after the yoga intervention.

One review of yoga and mindfulness after stroke has been completed (Lazaridou, Philbrook, and Tzika, 2013). There were few studies that included yoga and all have already been discussed here. Overall, the authors indicated that only a few studies have been completed and have all been relatively small and without active control groups. The authors do, however, conclude that yoga may be a valuable clinical intervention for clients with stroke and that, perhaps, yoga is something clients can be taught to do on their own to enhance their recovery.

Merging Yoga and Rehabilitation

We recognize that most therapists do not have the luxury of providing weekly hour-long sessions to their clients. From our research, it does appear that some rehabilitation facilities are beginning to offer an hour-long yoga session a week, but most therapists are having to merge yoga with their ongoing rehabilitation time with their clients. But our own research has shown us that it may be best when we add yoga to therapy. For example, as already discussed, we added yoga to ongoing inpatient rehabilitation and found that participants and therapists thought that the yoga enhanced recovery after an acute event (Schmid, *et al.*, 2014; Van Puymbroeck, *et al.*, 2015).

More recently, we developed and tested a new intervention, called Merging Yoga and Occupational Therapy (MY-OT) (Schmid, *et al.*, 2016b). We found that, after yoga, our clients had significant improvements in balance, strength, range of motion, and confidence to not fall (Schmid, *et al.*, 2012), but we quickly realized that they also needed some education about their "new body and abilities" and about preventing future falls. For example, one client had such improved balance that he climbed a ladder and got on to his roof to clean out the gutters! We were excited to hear about these increased activities, but very concerned about someone with hemiparesis and other stroke-related disabilities climbing on to the roof! We then developed a group occupational therapy intervention that was focused on fall prevention and fall risk factor modification (Schmid, *et al.*, 2015c). The group occupational therapy included identification and management of fall risk factors in the environment. When we paired yoga with the group occupational therapy intervention, we found improvements in balance, balance confidence, and risk factor management (Atler, *et al.*, 2017; Portz, *et al.*, 2016; Schmid, *et al.*, 2016b). Due to the success of the MY-OT program, we are now preparing to trial interventions where we merge yoga and other therapy in multiple other diagnostic populations, such as for clients with cancer or diabetes.

Summary

In summary, we recommend that yoga and rehabilitation therapists include yoga as they can into their treatment and that yoga may enhance therapeutic outcomes, including progress and recovery, for clients who have a stroke. The addition of yoga to clinical practice will look different for different types of therapists. We therefore also recommend that the therapist follows their national practice framework or their local scope of practice when available.

CHAPTER 5

Incorporating the Therapeutic Practice of Yoga After Stroke

Yoga as a Pathway in Post-Stroke Rehabilitation

In this chapter, we briefly review key considerations and suggestions for incorporating yoga into post-stroke rehabilitation. For those therapists who really want to integrate yoga into practice, we recommend completing a yoga teacher training to be more fully immersed in yoga teachings. This book is written for therapists, including yoga therapists, who want to include yoga during rehabilitation for clients with stroke. We include pathways to do this, modifications for yoga poses, case studies, and other resources. We fully believe that yoga is both feasible and beneficial after stroke. It is, however, up to the therapist to: fully understand the client's medical history; make decisions regarding use of group yoga or one-to-one yoga; be able to modify poses; integrate yoga into daily activities; and always maintain the safety of the client. We must listen to our clients to best understand their needs to facilitate their growth and recovery after stroke.

As we move into discussing the use of yoga in rehabilitation practice, it is important to review some basic physiology. The nervous system includes the central nervous system and the peripheral nervous system. The central nervous system includes the brain and spinal cord. The peripheral nervous system includes the peripheral nerves, muscles, and neuromuscular junctions. The peripheral nervous system is then also divided into the autonomic nervous system and the somatic nervous system. The autonomic nervous system controls the vital organs—the heart, liver, intestines, and other internal organs—and is therefore responsible for involuntary organ function. Most functions of the autonomic nervous system are involuntary and include the visceral innervations. The autonomic nervous system has two branches: the sympathetic nervous system and the parasympathetic nervous system. Typically, if there is activity in the sympathetic nervous system, the parasympathetic nervous system has less activity or vice versa. When the sympathetic nervous system is activated, the body is equipped to deal with an emergency. The body releases stress hormones such as cortisol and adrenaline, and increases blood pressure, heart rate, and oxygen and blood flow to the large muscles of the body. These changes enable the person to be ready for "fight or flight" in the face of the stressor. On the other hand, the parasympathetic nervous system is restorative in nature or "rest and digest."

When the parasympathetic nervous system is activated, blood pressure is reduced, blood flow returns to the rest of the body, and the body quiets. Yoga can target both the sympathetic nervous system and parasympathetic nervous system. Active practices like sun salutations activate the sympathetic nervous system, while restorative yoga poses and meditation activate the parasympathetic nervous system.

The somatic nervous system is the other part of the peripheral system and is associated with voluntary movement or control of the skeletal muscles. The somatic nervous system is made up of the afferent or sensory nerves and efferent or motor nerves. The afferent or sensory nerves transmit feelings of sensation to the central nervous system from the body. The efferent or motor nerves provide demands from the central nervous system to the body, such as muscle contraction.

Because of its versatility, yoga is a great tool for rehabilitation and yoga therapists to use for individuals with stroke to enhance recovery in the acute, rehabilitative, and chronic stages of recovery. This chapter reviews some key considerations for using yoga with this population, including contraindications, precautions, and considerations for including yoga in therapy. We will also cover modifications and props for making yoga accessible for everyone that may help the individual move deeper into the pose; see Chapter 6 for recommended postures (asanas) using the floor, chair, and standing.

Contraindications for Yoga with Individuals with Stroke

In order to safely include yoga as part of post-stroke rehabilitation, the therapist should consider and address multiple contraindications for yoga with individuals with stroke.

- Inversions are contraindicated for high blood pressure and for people with a recent stroke because of the increased blood flow to the brain that results from the inverted posture.

- Individuals with acute or recent stroke should avoid all poses where the head drops below the waist because of increased blood flow to the brain. If blood pressure is well controlled, and the person is in the chronic stages of stroke recovery, inversions may be considered, cautiously.

- Modify all standing poses by not bending forward further than the torso parallel to the floor. You can use wall modifications, such as teaching Half Downward Facing Dog (Ardha Adho Mukha Svanasana) at the wall.

- Avoid breath retention (kumbhaka) in the acute stages of stroke recovery, as well as in the chronic stages if blood pressure is high.

Precautions for Yoga with Individuals with Stroke

As we've described previously, a stroke may change the ability of an individual to engage in physical activity, or it may introduce new things to take into consideration prior to engaging in physical activity. Below we outline some precautions to keep in mind prior to engaging the client with stroke in yoga.

- If dizziness occurs in a supine position, prop the individual's head to reduce dizziness.

- After a stroke, an individual may experience orthostatic hypotension—a swift decrease in blood pressure upon standing. It is very important to be conscientious about this and stand in proximity to your client in order to catch them if there is a loss of balance upon standing.

- Blood pressure may also still be high or uncontrolled after stroke. Until it is controlled, it is important to assess and manage the client's current blood pressure before implementing any intervention. In our research studies, we take everyone's blood pressure immediately prior to the session beginning. If the blood pressure is >190/90, we ask the participant not to proceed with the class but to listen to the class and think about moving through the postures (mental practice). If the blood pressure is >160/79 but <190/90 we will give the participant a choice between completing class or resting. We encourage the individual to sit and relax until it lowers. This is a good time to practice some pranayama or dhyana techniques. We also reassess blood pressure before transitioning to standing or floor work. If blood pressure increases to >190/90 we do not allow participants to transition to standing or floor work, and we recommend they contact their physician immediately.

- Assess allergies. Most yoga mats are latex, and a latex-free yoga mat will need to be provided for individuals with latex allergies. We have also had clients who are allergic to specific scents, so the use of scented essential oils in eye pillows or in the room will also need to be evaluated for suitability for the specific client.

Additional Considerations for Yoga with Individuals with Stroke

- Consider having clients with stroke practice flat on their backs if they are able to transfer to the floor or mat table—the therapist can recreate or modify most poses for prone or supine positioning.

- Because balance and equilibrium are challenged or different after stroke, initial forays into yoga practice can occur in bed, with a transition to a chair, a mat table, or the floor when the client is ready.

- Stay close for hands-on assists if needed until you are comfortable with the individual's balance, in both seated or standing poses.

- Because some strokes are caused by plaque being released from an artery and subsequently lodging in the brain, it is important to avoid twisting the carotid artery, as this is the primary source of blood for the brain. Dr. Baxter Bell (2007) recommends avoiding twisting the neck and having the belly and chest create the twist instead of the neck. He also recommends a focus on elongating the neck and maintaining a soft front of the throat. Another option is to keep the head in the same plane as the body or in a comfortable, neutral position.

- Use a wall, chair, or mat table for additional support. All yoga postures can be done sitting in a chair. Use props to reduce any strain!

- Evaluate what time of day works best for your clients—their abilities and energy may differ from morning to afternoon.

- A common refrain in yoga is to listen to one's body. This is also important as part of rehabilitation; encourage the individual to listen to their body, push themselves towards their edge, and move past it where possible during yoga practice. However, reduced or different sensations after stroke may not provide the same cues to the individual as they did previously. Therefore, the therapist should encourage the client to recognize tingling, heat, or unusual feelings as potential sensations of discomfort.

- It is important to consider adding contralateral movements and incorporating them into yoga postures. These are movements in which muscles on the opposite sides of the body are exercised simultaneously. These movements are thought to activate both hemispheres of the brain and should be included in yoga poses to facilitate that activation. There are several suggestions of where this could be added into the poses listed in Chapter 6.

Yoga Is Not "No Pain No Gain"

Yoga may be therapeutic for people and even life changing for some. Once a person begins a yoga practice and begins to feel the benefits of yoga, they often report changes in cognitive, emotional, and physical aspects of their body. However, while yoga may become everything to some people, it may not be as relevant for others. For some individuals, yoga may simply be a physical activity or a way to improve the physical body. As therapists, we must be able to accept this and be client centered, allowing the client to know what they need and to what level they are able to accept yoga into their current lives. One reason that yoga is often so easily accepted by our clients with chronic stroke is that they have tried everything else; they are willing to try something new, as they are frustrated with their current state of being. While yoga may be therapeutic and used as an important aspect of therapy, it is important to note that clients may be willing to use yoga as it is not painful. Sometimes, during typical post-stroke rehabilitation, there is a "no pain no gain" mentality; however, this cannot be true during a yoga practice. We hope that yoga helps a person feel more and be more in tune with their own body, but we do not push a person into yoga postures to a point where there is pain.

More often in yoga, we attempt to come to the "edge," and we sometimes try to move beyond the edge. Coming to the edge or meeting the edge means that the client begins to come to a place where their mind and/or body begins to feel a resistance or a challenge. As therapists, we must help the clients understand when it is time to stay at the edge and when it is time to begin to move beyond the edge. If at any time the client is feeling pain, it is time to back off. In a yoga practice, there are a few ways to facilitate the client moving beyond the edge and into the resistance or the challenge, whether to the mind or body. Remember to not create pain or bring your client harm—teach the client to be considerate of their own edge, remembering the yama of ahimsa (non-harming). Always remind clients to listen to and honor their bodies and to know that where they are is enough. Consider the following when helping your client with stroke meet, and then safely move beyond, their edge.

- **Maintain the yoga pose**: If the client is not feeling pain or discomfort, then help them stay in the pose. Remember that people with stroke may have decreased sensation and thus may not be able to feel pain or discomfort, but they can still injure themselves. The therapist must be aware of this to not cause harm, pain, or injury (ahimsa).

- **Breathe into the yoga pose**: As always, we connect the breath to the movement in yoga. When in the pose and at the edge, or trying to move past the edge, ask the client to take deep breaths to calm the mind and the body. Often, the deep exhale also allows space for additional movement or flexibility. If the client cannot take long smooth breaths while in a posture, it is time to back off and not push as hard.

- **Contract and relax the muscles while in the yoga pose**: It is a common form of neuro-reeducation to contract and relax muscles and to contract muscles, relax, and then push a little more (or have the therapist resist the client's movement). This use of neuro-reeducation can also be used during yoga with your client. While in a yoga pose ask the client to contract and then relax the muscles. This technique will help the client move a little deeper into the pose. If the client is not able to relax the muscles, they should be asked to back off from the pose.

Yoga Helps to Be in the Moment and More Accepting After a Stroke

Yoga makes us more mindful, and thoughtful, about other important areas of our lives or our lifestyle. This is true for people who have sustained stroke, as well. Yoga after stroke may help people make other healthier decisions, for example be more mindful or thoughtful about food choices. Through yoga, people may be "more in the moment," not worrying about the past or the present. When people are living their day-to-day lives more in the current moment, they may make better choices or be more cognizant of their surrounds. For example, we have heard from multiple clients in our yoga studies that yoga helped them focus more on their current body and surroundings and therefore helped in reducing falls and injuries. This occurred simply through living in the moment and being less distracted. In one of our studies with veterans who had sustained a stroke at least six months prior to the study, a man named Sean compared how his life was different following the yoga intervention with before. He stated:

> Well, I remember first getting home from the hospital and starting stuff, like walking on my own and doing stuff around the house. Again, I would get so anxious and so nervous about stuff…you know…how am I going to do that. I think with this program that doesn't even enter into it anymore. (Van Puymbroeck *et al.*, 2014, p.26)

Making Yoga Accessible for Everyone

Props are a great way to make yoga postures available for everyone. Almost any pose can be modified with the use of a prop. The most common props are a wall, chair with a back and without wheels, bolsters, straps, blocks, blankets, sand bags, and eye pillows. The rehabilitation environment also offers the possibility of a mat table as a great prop.

- A wall can be very helpful and supportive for your client. It can assist with standing postures by providing a strong support to reduce falls.

- Chairs with backs provide a vehicle for individuals to participate in a posture without concerns of falling. Arm rests are also necessary for clients with impaired balance. In more chronic stroke, chairs without arm rests may be appropriate. Make sure to use chairs that do not have wheels on the feet.

- Bolsters can be rectangular, flat, or round, and can vary in diameter. Bolsters are similar to foam rollers but are softer and provide support, particularly in restorative poses.

- Yoga straps help to elongate reach. They are typically about six feet long and may include a buckle at one end so that loops can be made in the strap. Gait belts can easily double as a yoga strap.

- Blocks are typically wood, rubber, or cork. Blocks can be used under hands or feet to bring the ground closer. Blocks can be used at three levels—short, medium, and tall—and can be used to progressively make tasks more difficult by changing the height of the block.

- Blankets can be used to make a softer or slightly higher seat, provide comfort for the head or neck, and as a covering during restorative postures.

- Sandbags can be filled with 5–15 pounds of sand and then used as a means to weight an extremity or the torso. Applying a sandbag to a spastic limb may help to relax that limb; however, be careful to not place a sandbag where it may cause injury if the client cannot sense the injury or pain secondary to sensory impairment.

- In our research studies, we have found that most individuals enjoy using an eye pillow. Eye pillows are usually filled with a grain and may be infused with an essential oil, such as lavender. These are typically used in the final resting pose, Corpse pose (Savasana).

- In the rehabilitation environment, a mat table may also be available. We have used mat tables in our research for individuals who were not able to move to the ground for supine work or were not comfortable with the idea of doing this. Mat tables offer a possibility for additional work by bringing a flat and safe surface closer to the individual. Mat tables also provide a stable surface to fold towards in any type of forward fold.

- It is important for the rehabilitation therapist to pay close attention to the posture of the client. Oftentimes after a stroke, posture is slumped forward or to one side. The rehabilitation therapist should encourage Axial Extension (Rekha) (sitting up straight). Directions on how to do this are in Chapter 6.

In addition to props, the therapist should use verbal and tactile cueing to provide both visual and auditory cues for the individual. Remember that individuals with stroke may have receptive impairments, so keeping verbal cues short and sweet is important. The therapist may also need to provide hands-on or visual support for the hemiparetic side so that clients can engage in movements that require bilateral engagement to the extent possible.

Proper Mechanics for Stroke Care

It is very common that people with hemiplegia forget to attend to the side of the body that has hemiplegia; however, we know the following from research related to neuroplasticity.

- Activating the neuroplasticity in the brain can help the brain to heal. When neuroplasticity is activated, the brain begins to form new neural connections.

- Repetition is key to activating neuroplasticity. Therefore, it is important to repeat practices and to use the hemiplegic side of the body, even if the limbs need to be assisted through the asanas. Research indicates that more repetitions of each task result in better responses, so do not hesitate to ask your client to engage in a number of repetitions (Carey, et al., 2002; Liepert, et al., 1998).

People with hemiplegia may also have hemi-spatial neglect—meaning that they ignore the paralyzed side of the body—so proper body mechanics are really important during recovery, including during yoga. For people with hemi-spatial neglect, positioning is important to increase stimulation of the neglected side. This can include providing tactile input and stimulation to the neglected limbs as well as environmental stimulation on the neglected side.

When seated, the individual with hemi-spatial neglect or hemiparesis should be in a non-moving chair with a firm back and bilateral arm rests. The therapist will want to assess the client's upright orientation. If the client's feet cannot reach the floor, place a yoga block or foot stool underneath the feet so that their feet are not just hanging unsupported. If the client is leaning to one side, the therapist can adjust the seat so that there are supports (such as a bolster) to encourage an upright posture. The affected or paralyzed arm should be supported on an adjustable base with a pillow or blanket underneath. There should be equal weight on both buttocks, and the feet should rest flat on the floor (or support). If the client is lying down flat on their back, the affected arm should be supported with a pillow.

It is very important to perform transfers to the non-neglected side. Gait belts are very helpful and should be placed around the client's waist while the client is sitting on the edge of the bed. Remember to place your hands on the gait belt, block the hemiparetic knee, and allow the client's trunk and knees to move forward during the transfer. Avoid pulling the client's affected arm when transferring. Remember to keep a wide base of support, stand close to the client, maintain a neutral spine and flexion in your lower body, and shift your weight with the client's movement.

Some additional handling ideas for working with individuals who have had stroke include: using an open hand; adding pressure in the assists slowly; and moving slowly and cautiously. It is also important for yoga postures to be held for at least 30 seconds. Finally, encourage weight bearing on the affected side and involvement of the affected arm.

Yoga in Acute Care

In the time immediately following a stroke, a person may be seen in acute care by a therapist during the stabilization period. See Chapter 12 for sample yoga practices in the acute setting. During this time, there is a lot of sitting and waiting for the next treatment or procedure, while also trying to sort out the myriad of emotions that accompany a stroke. Loved ones are also around and may not have ideas of what to do or expect. Involving the caregiver in some gentle yoga practice is a kind act, as they can also appreciate the benefits that accompany a yoga practice. See Chapter 13 for additional information about the caregiver and yoga. When a stroke occurs, the client may not be able to control their body or movements, and their mind may become disconnected from the body. Teaching pranayama (breath work) can help a person reconnect with their body, help them to feel in control of their body, and may help them reduce their fears associated with the stroke or stroke-related disability. Pranayama helps to enhance focus and clarity in the mind, increases calm, and balances the oxygen and carbon dioxide levels in the body. In pranayama practices, we learn to focus on the breath, inhale deeply, exhale slowly, and experience positive emotions associated with the release of breath. Breath helps to coordinate the mind and body, so pranayama is helpful in advancing stroke recovery.

Mental practice may be a great way to make yoga accessible to individuals in acute care (and in rehabilitation), in addition to enhancing recovery. Mental practice is the repetitious cognitive rehearsal of specific physical movements, such as yoga postures. Mental practice is very useful for a number of reasons: it does not require any physical ability or practice; it can be completed without a therapist or teacher present; and it does not require any cost or equipment. According to Dr. Stephen Page and Heather Peters (2014), there are a few keys to mental practice for individuals who are post-stroke:

- Mental practice is most successful when paired with the execution of the corresponding physical skill. Mental practice combined with rehabilitation results in more functioning than mental practice alone. However, mental practice on its own has also demonstrated some improvements in functioning. Furthermore, the researchers reported that there are higher levels of generalization to unique environments when clients with stroke pair mental and physical practice.

- Mental practice typically begins with listening to an audio recording through headphones for approximately 30 minutes. The recording includes:

  - a warm up that encourages the client to think about a warm place and to engage in progressive muscle relaxation by contracting and relaxing the muscles (for three to five minutes)

  - mental rehearsal of the physical practice that happened that day; several trials for each of the physical tasks are practiced mentally (for 20 minutes)

  - relaxation and refocusing (for three to five minutes).

So, to translate this evidence into acute care, therapists can start the yoga practice with a few key asanas (poses) and then provide a recording that describes these asanas in enough detail that the individual can imagine themselves doing them. Page and Peters also encourage the use of PRACTICE principles for neurorehabilitation and mental practice, described below in relation to incorporating into yoga practice in acute care.

- **P**art-whole practice should be used: Activity analysis principles should be applied to the asanas; that is, identify the required components for each asana. Repeat the execution of the smaller components, as well as practicing the entire task.

- **R**epetitive and goal focused: The affected body parts should be used in the repetitive practice of the specific asana.

- **A**ctivities should be meaningful: Asanas should be discussed in terms of their benefit to the individual *and* should be related to something that is meaningful for the individual. Think strength, stress relief, activating the neural pathways, and so forth.

- **C**lient-driven: Encourage the client to identify directions for therapy and asanas when appropriate.

- **T**rain in a practical way: Choose asanas that are easy to understand and follow, for both the person who is post-stroke and their family member. Consider giving a hand out with the practices that have been worked on together, so that the individual has a visual cue to use in mental practice or, if it is appropriate, for the individual to practice individually.

- **I**mpairments should be addressed: If impairments exist that limit participation, try to address them through choosing asanas and pranayama that will address these impairments. Also consider using mental practice to enhance the practice of working on these impairments.

- **C**hallenge regularly and appropriately: Make the yoga practice progressively more challenging. There are so many options for grading yoga asanas and pranayama. Identify ways to start with the least complicated and difficult version of the asana, and progress these as the individual's abilities improve.

- **E**mphasize accomplishments: Identify specific examples of improvements that the individual has made in yoga practice.

There may not be a lot of time or availability for an asana practice in acute care. A good and low-key asana for acute care is Simhasana (pronounced sim-ha-sana), or Lion's pose. This pose can be done seated in a chair or on a bed. This is thought to be one of the most robust facial exercises, as it involves many facial muscles working together. See Chapter 6 for instructions for the pose, but start the pose from sitting up straight instead of kneeling on the floor.

Yoga as a Treatment Intervention in Rehabilitation

Yoga is being infused into rehabilitation in many ways. Some rehabilitation centers are offering yoga via their rehabilitation therapists, and some are offering yoga as a stand-alone program for their clients and/or caregivers. Still others are offering yoga as part of support provided in support/extended care groups. We conducted a study where we added yoga to typical therapy in group or one-to-one yoga sessions. Rehabilitation clients identified that there were three primary areas of benefit from participating in yoga, including: breathing; relaxation; and psychological well-being (Schmid, *et al.*, 2015b). Research subjects identified that a focus on breathing helped them to feel more calm, as well as increasing their breathing capacity. They also identified that being able to breathe and focus on their breath during difficult or painful activities or interventions (including activities of daily living and mobility) made a substantial difference in being able to complete those tasks. They identified that the relaxation techniques from yoga also helped them feel more relaxed and less apprehensive. Research subjects also reported feeling less stress and anxiety and being more able to cope with their current health situation, as well as having a feeling of being in control of something during a time where they feel little control.

We also found support for yoga in the rehabilitation setting from an administrator and agency perspective (Van Puymbroeck, *et al.*, 2015). Rehabilitation therapists identified that having a yoga therapist administer yoga helped to provide holistic care to the clients, and this bridged the gap between physical, occupational, and recreational therapies. Administrators were also in support of yoga, as it helped with holistically addressing the mind, body, and spirit of their clients—something that was important to the mission of the hospitals.

Clients who sustain a stroke require relearning of some or many common behaviors. This requires neural reprogramming and adaptations in the brain tissue that allows this brain tissue to learn and take over the function of the lost neurons. We do not fully understand how this happens; however, we believe that information is re-routed and healthy brain tissue is reprogrammed. The process of reprogramming the brain is exhausting, both physically and mentally, for the individual, and they will need a lot of sleep. Therefore, it is important to incorporate both physically active and restorative sequences for your clients.

Asanas can start to be explored during inpatient rehabilitation and beyond. Asanas can help to connect hemispheres by including both sides of the body in poses to retrain neural pathways. Asanas can be done seated, standing, on a mat table, or on the floor. After a stroke, individuals may have difficulty distinguishing the left from the right side. It will be important that as you lead them through the sequence, you allow extra time for processing and provide visual demonstrations of the asanas.

Restorative yoga is a very different practice, with the primary intent being rest and restoration.

Restorative Yoga

As previously described, stroke recovery is exhausting, emotionally and physically. This means that the body and mind experience stress following a stroke, and yoga is well situated to help the body manage this stress. Restorative yoga can activate the parasympathetic nervous system and help the body with "rest and digest," or tapping into the relaxation response. Restorative yoga is just that—the opportunity to restore balance and peace into the body. Restorative poses are done seated or on the floor (or a mat table) in prone or supine position. In restorative yoga, many props are used to support the body to enhance and support the relaxation response.

Yoga for Vision Changes After Stroke

Although not as widely discussed as other stroke-related outcomes, vision may get worse following stroke. According to the Australian Stroke Association (2018), about one third of individuals have decreased vision following a stroke, and this vision is often not fully recovered. In our first yoga study for individuals with stroke, we were surprised by the three individuals with chronic stroke (at least five years post-stroke) who reported increased vision, which their neuro-ophthalmologist thought was likely due to practices such as Alternate Nostril Breathing (Nadi Shodhana Pranayama) which specifically targeted the bilateral hemispheres of the brain. We had not anticipated these changes, thus we did not measure vision, but we did record their comments about the vision changes. While these changes did not happen for everyone, we think it is important to briefly describe the changes that we think are related to yoga practice, including the yoga eye exercises that were included in each yoga session. We have not objectively measured vision, acuity, or reading in any of our studies; instead, we simply share subjective stories reported by a few of our study participants.

A man named Hugh, who had a stroke in his early 40s, was a participant in one of our studies. After the stroke, Hugh had lost his driver's license and was trying to improve his skills to be able to safely drive again. Hugh happened to go to the eye doctor before and after the eight-week yoga intervention and reported the changes to the study team. Before the yoga study, Hugh's vision was 20/400 (considered a severe impairment or severe low vision). After eight weeks of yoga that included the yoga eye exercises, Hugh reported that his vision improved to 20/40 (considered a mild vision loss, but close to normal vision). Hugh's ophthalmologist attributed these changes to yoga, specifically the vision exercise, but also the Alternate Nostril Breathing, which is thought to activate both hemispheres of the brain. The ophthalmologist thought that neuroplasticity allowed for the yoga to develop new pathways to allow for enhanced vision.

A woman named Cacia, who was in her mid-60s when she sustained a stroke, also participated in one of our studies; the study included the same yoga intervention as Hugh received. Towards the end of the study, after about six weeks of yoga, Cacia reported she noticed changes to her vision. After her stroke, but before yoga, Cacia was not able to read a white font written on a dark background. Cacia's best example of when she would see a white font on dark backgrounds was on car bumper stickers. She was not able to read the white font; instead the letters became swirled and confusing to her. On the way to yoga one day, as her husband was driving, she excitedly realized she could read a bumper sticker on the car in front of her. She reported this change to the study staff and continued to show improvement during the last two weeks of the study. Cacia and the team also attributed this change in her ability to read a white font to the yoga vision exercise performed during each yoga class.

Reduced vision after stroke is caused by one-sided damage to the brain affecting both eyes because the optic nerves travel together in the brain. Visual field loss, such as homonymous hemianopsia (loss of half of the visual field in each or one eye) and quadrantanopia (loss of vision in the upper or lower quarter of the visual field), may occur. Other visual issues include difficulties with eye movement (such as strabismus or diplopia) or unsteady movement, such as nystagmus. Following stroke, individuals may also experience an increase in dry eye and visual neglect.

Other damage in the brain may seem to impact vision, but the visual changes are actually related to what the brain perceives and how the brain interprets information. In this case, the eyes and neural pathways work correctly, but the brain does not correctly process the information. When this happens, the client is diagnosed with *visual agnosia* and cannot recognize familiar objects or people's faces. The client may also develop a *visual neglect*, where they will not be able to respond to things, or even be aware of things, on the affected side of the body.

Stroke-related vision changes may be significant and will be frustrating for the client and the family. Some natural recovery may occur after the stroke. The therapist must take compromised vision into account when treating the client. If the client has a visual neglect, they will not see the therapist approach from the side that is affected and are at risk for being startled.

Due to these visual outcomes from stroke, rehabilitation therapists may elect to include asanas for the eyes. The Sivananda tradition offers several specific eye asanas (Ruiz, 2007). To instruct this sequence:

1. Invite the client to start in Corpse pose (Savasana) to relax or to start in a relaxed seated pose in a chair or on the mat table.

2. After a short period in Corpse pose (Savasana), have the client transition to sit in Easy pose (Sukhasana). Suggest that they keep their eyes open and body relaxed and maintain the stillness of the head and neck. In our previous studies, we found that some individuals felt nauseous keeping their eyes open. If this is the case, the individual can close their eyes for this practice.

3. Ask the client to:

   i. imagine a clock in front of their eyes

   ii. raise their eyes to 12:00; hold for one second

   iii. lower their eyes to 6:00; hold for one second

   iv. continue to raise and lower their eyes for ten repetitions, without blinking if able

   v. Keep the gaze straight ahead and relaxed.

4. After the ten repetitions, instruct the client to quickly rub their palms together to warm them up and place them in a cupping motion over each eye, without

pressure. This encourages the eyes to relax in the darkness. Suggest to the client that they may be able to feel the warm energy (prana) from their hands after rubbing them together.

5. Prepare your client for another round of eye movements, by instructing the following:

   i.   now, picturing the clock again, move the eyes to 9:00; hold for one second

   ii. move the eyes to 3:00; hold for one second

   iii. picture 2:00; hold for one second

   iv. picture 7:00; hold for one second.

6. Repeat ten times, and then cup the eyes again as in Step 4.

7. Prepare your client for another round of eye movements, by instructing the following:

   i.   picture 11:00; hold for one second

   ii. picture 4:00; hold for one second.

8. Repeat ten times, and then cup the eyes again as in Step 4.

9. Conclude the practice with ten full eye circles around the clock in each direction—clockwise and counterclockwise.

Mudras

Mudras can simultaneously calm the mind and engage those with limited function. Mudras are hand positions, also considered gestures or seals, that help to channel the body's energy flow and the internal journey. Mudras are most often used during meditation or pranayama to encourage the flow of energy in the body—this is how the internal journey becomes more intentional. Eastern medicine practitioners believe that the different areas of the hands are connected with parts of the body and the brain; thus when parts of the hands are stimulated, the corresponding hand and brain regions are activated, leading to a specific state of mind. See Chapter 10 for a description of the meanings associated with the hands and for the most popular mudras.

Mantras

A mantra is a word or phrase that is repeated. It is thought that mantras make the mind strong and clearly focused on the message of the mantra, and, over time, the message becomes embedded in the mind and the mind becomes still. When the mind becomes still, so many benefits can occur, particularly for individuals who are post-stroke who may be flooded with competing thoughts or simply have clouded thinking because of the effort required in recovery. The use of mantras may be particularly helpful for clients with communication issues, such as aphasia.

Clients with stroke often do not feel whole, or they lament the person they "used to be." We have found mantras to be helpful in the healing process. Mantras appropriate for stroke recovery include:

- "I am strong enough."

- "I am whole enough."

- "I am enough."

If you want to use mantras to help the individual visualize the chakras or the properties associated with the chakras, the following mantras may be appropriate:

- Root chakra: "I am safe." "I am strong and I am stable."

- Sacral chakra: "I am well and I have enough." "I am creative."

- Solar plexus chakra: "I am enough."

- Heart chakra: "I am loved." "I have compassion for myself and others."

- Throat chakra: "I am heard." "I can express myself."

- Third eye chakra: "My mind is calm." "My mind is open to new ideas."

- Crown chakra: "I surrender to what I do not know or do not understand."

- Aura chakra: "I am strong, I am healthy, I am vibrant."

Some traditional mantras that are used in yoga classes include the following.

- **Om/Aum**: This is the original sound current, or the sound of the universe. This can be said once or several times. Om/Aum is an affirmation of the universal, divine presence. It is thought that chanting Om helps the individual on the path towards wholeness and higher consciousness.

- **Lokah Samastha**: This mantra is one for wholeness, and the full mantra is: Lokah samastha sukhino bhavanthu (pronounced ow-kaah'-ha suh-muh-staah'-ha soo-khee-no' buh'-fun-too). This translates roughly to "May this world be established with a sense of well-being and happiness."

- **Om Shanti Shanti Shanti**: The Sanskrit term shanti translates to "peace," "bliss," or "calm." This mantra represents peace in the mind, peace in speech, and peace in the physical body. It can be used as a greeting or end-of-class salutation.

- **Sat Nam**: Pronounced "sut naam," this Gurmukhi mantra from the Kundalini yoga tradition translates to "Truth is my name." It is used as a greeting, a closing, and a mantra for centering.

- **Ra Ma Da Sa Sa Say So Hung**: This is also a Gurmukhi mantra from the Kundalini yoga tradition that can be used as a restorative mantra to send healing to the self and to others. It translates to "Sun, Moon, Earth, Infinity, All that is in infinity, I am thee."

Chanting

Chanting could be a great opportunity for co-treatment with the speech therapist on your rehabilitation team. Chanting helps individuals to feel the vibration of the word that is being chanted throughout the body and can help with speech functions. Chanting can help to balance the left and right sides of the brain (through the ida and pingala nadis—the energy channels that are thought to spiral around the spine like a double helix of our DNA). Chanting Om/Aum in acute stages of recovery may be a technique to help the individual bring awareness to the areas of the body, thus increasing neural connections. Chanting can be considered very therapeutic; it opens the heart of the chanter to a connection with the Divine energy. Just as music is a very therapeutic modality, chanting can be a very therapeutic part of a yoga intervention. Any of the above mantras can be chanted audibly.

Chanting can also be done as a song and accompanied by music. This may help the individual feel less self-conscious about saying or singing words out loud. One positive and uplifting chant comes from the Kundalini tradition and is often used as the final song of a practice. The song is called the "Long Time Sun Shine" song, and there are many musical variations available. The lyrics are: "May the long time sun shine upon you, all love surround you, and the pure light within you, guide your way on. Sat nam."

Meditation (Dhyana)

Meditation can be helpful in managing the stress and uncertainty that comes with stroke. Yoga Nidra may be helpful, with a focus on the parts of the body that have been affected. Yoga Nidra is considered yogic sleep, and it is believed that one hour of Yoga Nidra is equal to four hours of deep sleep. Some of the benefits associated with Yoga Nidra include: deep relaxation; balancing the nervous system and increased production of endorphins; stress relief and reduction in depression, anxiety, and pain; and increased clarity of thought. You, as the rehabilitation therapist or the person wanting to practice Yoga Nidra, can modify the script to the specific situation. See Chapter 9 for a Yoga Nidra script written specifically for this population of clients with stroke. Also in Chapter 9 you will find directions for Kirtan Kriya. Kirtan Kriya is a multifactorial meditation and combines chanting, mudras, and drishti (gazing point).

CHAPTER 6

Descriptions and Modifications of Asanas (Postures) for Yoga Post-Stroke

Introduction to Asanas (Postures)

The asanas, or postures, contained in this chapter are those that have been used in yoga studies for people with stroke or are identified in the case studies found in Chapter 11 or in sample practices in Chapter 12. Postures are listed in alphabetical order by their English or common name, and the Sanskrit name is also provided. Benefits of each posture are included, and modifications are noted for each posture. The modifications identified are suggestions, but the therapist should feel free to modify poses beyond what is suggested here. We suggest that you use props and materials in your environment to make asanas fully available to your patient. We also provide pictures of these poses in seated, standing, and wall versions (as available) to provide visual understanding of these asanas. Note that these asanas are described without modification to the traditional pose, but that in yoga for individuals with stroke, these postures can be modified using the suggestion provided.

Some translations that help with understanding the Sanskrit terms are given here.

- Apana: downward-flowing life force.

- Ardha: half.

- Asana: pose.

- Drishti: focus of the eyes.

- Eka: one.

- Pada: leg or foot.

- Prana: vital life force.

- Salamba: with support.

- Supta: supine.

- Tan: to stretch or extend.

- Ut: intense.

- Uttiha: extended.

Please note: The information compiled here is from widely available sources. We have taken care to report information accurately and fully; however, as with any physical activity, there are risks inherent in moving the body. The precautions and contra-indications noted are drawn from a variety of sources. The lack of a precaution or contraindication does not guarantee its safety nor is it all encompassing. A number of poses identify that a precaution or contraindication is high blood pressure, something that may be an issue for an individual post-stroke, especially during the acute phases of post-stroke recovery. Consider grading the activities to make the appropriate modifications for your client using your clinical judgment. Furthermore, a teacher of ours, Lakshmi Voelker, used an approach to teaching chair yoga that is appropriate and applicable to all yoga poses and will make great sense to rehabilitation therapists. She recommends that there be three or more versions of each asana offered (such as Level 1, 2, or 3; or Option A, B, or C), so that individuals can choose the level of the pose that works best for them. These choices extend to both upper and lower body postures. Postures below are described in the typical interpretation of the pose, so therapists are encouraged to develop a yoga practice that is deep enough that they are able to identify three levels for each posture. Most of the seated or supine postures or modifications would be most accessible to your client if performed on a mat table instead of the floor.

Ankle Movements/Foot Flexion and Extension

This movement (see Figures 6.1 and 6.2) helps lubricate the joints and maintain range of motion in the joints. It can help clients with stroke improve proprioception and improve motor control in the lower extremities, including ankle and foot extension and flexion.

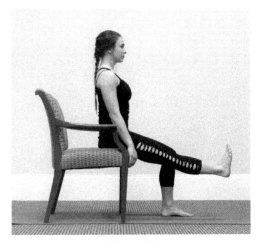

Figure 6.1

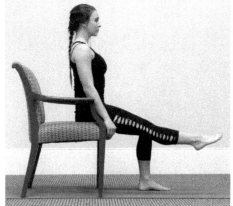

Figure 6.2

Precautions

No contraindications are noted.

Directions

1. Direct the client to begin in Axial Extension or Staff pose (Rekha).

2. On an exhale, they should flex the foot, drawing the toes back towards the leg.

3. On the inhale, they should extend the foot, pointing the toes away closer to the floor.

4. Ask them to repeat Steps 2 and 3.

Modifications/Props

• This can be done in any seat, including on the ground.

Anterior and Posterior Hip Tilts

This movement (see Figures 6.3 and 6.4) can be beneficial for improving proprioception and helping to improve hip and spinal alignment.

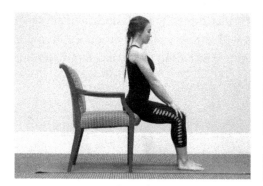

Figure 6.3

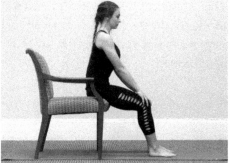

Figure 6.4

Precautions

No contraindications are noted for this movement.

Directions

1. This can be done seated on the ground or in a chair. Direct the client to begin in Easy pose (Sukhasana).

2. On the inhale, they should rock slightly forward on the hip bones, slightly arching the lower back and tilting the hips forward.

3. On the exhale, they should round the back and rock back on the sit bones, tilting the pelvis forward.

4. Ask them to repeat Steps 2 and 3.

Modifications/Props

- This can be done from supine, starting in Bridge pose, lowering the hips to the ground, and beginning hip tilts.

- This can also be modified to a standing pose by holding on to the wall or a chair and tilting the hips with each inhale and exhale.

Many of the above postures are typically completed standing but can be modified for a chair or floor practice. These asanas have the intent of building strength and flexibility of the upper and lower limbs.

Axial Extension or Staff Pose (Rekha)

Axial Extension or Staff pose (Rekha) (see Figure 6.5) helps to engage the core and encourage a strong seated posture. Sitting with a straight spine is important for good posture, something that is often diminished following stroke. It is completed in a chair in the provided sample practices in Chapter 12.

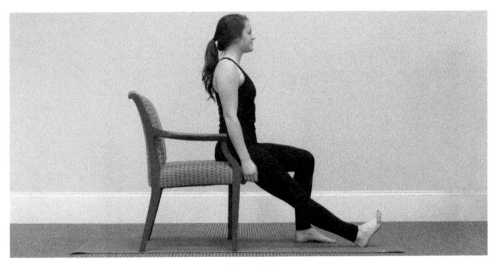

Figure 6.5

Precautions

None noted. The therapist and client must feel safe and may need to monitor blood pressure for orthostatic hypotension.

Directions

1. Direct the client to it, with the back straight, and the head gazing straight ahead. They should imagine extending the head towards the ceiling.

2. They should bring the shoulders up and roll the shoulder blades down the back.

3. They should extend both legs and imagine pressing the heels of the feet into the wall in front.

Modifications/Props

- Depending on leaning or slouching of the individual, blankets or bolsters can be used to provide tactile cues to elongate the spine.

- When this is done from a chair, blocks can be placed under the feet to bring the floor closer to the individual and provide support.

- Sitting on a blanket may reduce discomfort and help with proper alignment in the hips.

- To include contralateral movement, the movement of one arm and the opposite leg (or finger and thumb) can be incorporated.

Big Toe Pose (Padangusthasana)

Big Toe pose (Padangusthasana) (see Figure 6.6) is a forward fold, which is thought to stretch the back of the legs (hamstrings and calves) and the front of the legs (quadriceps). Big Toe pose (Padangusthasana) also calms the mind, reduces stress and anxiety, improves digestion, and may help to relieve headaches and insomnia.

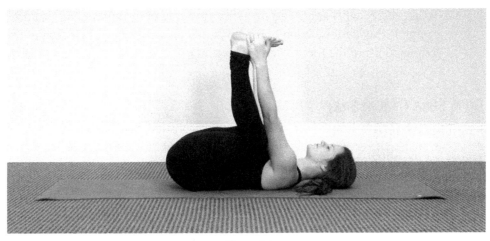

Figure 6.6

Precautions

This is a folding posture, so the full pose should not be done in the acute stages of stroke recovery or with individuals with high blood pressure. It should be used with caution with individuals with osteoporosis.

Directions

1. Direct the client to stand in Mountain pose (Tadasana) with the feet hip width apart. Ask them to inhale and contract the quadriceps to lift the knees. Next they should exhale, bend the knees slightly, and bend forward from the hips.

2. The head should hang in line with the torso. They should extend the arms and wrap the index and middle fingers around the big toes of each foot. They should tighten the grip and hold the toes securely and press the toes against the fingers.

3. They should inhale and lift the torso as much as possible while maintaining contact with the toes and raise the head with the torso. Next, they exhale and fold forward again, keeping the fingers wrapped around the toes.

4. Direct the client to repeat and release after several trials. They should bend the knees, bring the hands to the hips, and bring the torso upright.

Modifications/Props

- A yoga strap or gait belt can extend the reach. Loop the strap or gait belt under the arch of each foot, instead of holding on to the big toes. If the belt is held by the hand opposite to the extended leg, this is a contralateral exercise.

- To get the benefits and avoid dizziness that may occur in standing position, complete this pose by lying supine, wrapping a strap or gait belt around the foot and raising the foot towards the ceiling.

Boat Pose (Navasana)

Boat pose (Navasana) (see Figure 6.7) is a supine posture that has many levels of variation, making it very accessible for individuals of all ability levels. Some benefits of Boat pose (Navasana) include strengthening the belly and hip flexors and improving alignment of the spine, improving digestion, and stimulating the intestines, kidneys, and the thyroid and prostate glands. Boat pose (Navasana) also helps to reduce stress.

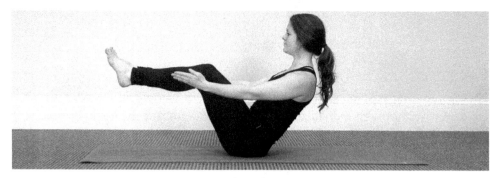

Figure 6.7

Precautions

There are a number of precautions or contraindications for Boat pose (Navasana). They include: asthma; diarrhea; headache; heart problems; insomnia; and low blood pressure. An individual with a neck injury should be positioned so that the head can rest on the wall while the torso is tilted.

Directions

1. Direct the client to sit on the floor with the knees bent and both feet flat on the floor.

2. They should place the hands on the ground behind the buttocks.

3. They should lift the spine and chest simultaneously, while leaning back slightly. Ask them to keep the spine straight.

4. While maintaining a straight spine, they should continue to lean back until seated on the sit bones and tailbone.

5. They should lift one foot and then the other off the floor, so that the calves are parallel to the floor, and ensure that the spine is straight and the chest is raised.

6. If available, they could try extending the legs until they are straight.

7. If possible, they could lift the arms from the ground and extend both arms with the thumbs facing the ceiling.

8. Direct the client to gently release the legs and arms.

Modifications/Props

- Sit in a chair at the end of the seat with the knees at right angles (see Figure 6.8). Hold the sides of the chair. Lean forward slightly and then tip back, lifting the feet off the floor.

- Perform a one-legged version of Boat pose (Navasana)—that is, with one foot raised at a time (see Figure 6.9). This can be made a contralateral exercise if the opposite arm is raised at the same time as the raised leg.

- Use a strap or gait belt to extend the reach of the hands or to loop around the arch of each foot to assist with balance (see Figure 6.10). Keeping the strap or belt taut is important.

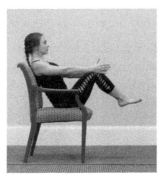 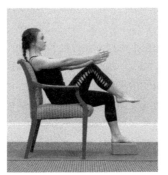 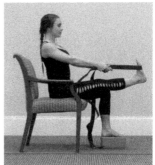

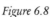

Figure 6.8   Figure 6.9   Figure 6.10

Bridge Pose (Setu Bandha Sarvangasana)

Bridge pose (Setu Bandha Sarvangasana) (see Figure 6.11) is done in supine position and stretches the chest, neck, and spine. It is thought to bring calm to the mind, reduce stress, and enhance mood. Bridge pose (Setu Bandha Sarvangasana) is also thought to help with digestion, stimulate the belly and associated organs, reduce pain such as headache and backache, and improve anxiety and fatigue. Bridge pose (Setu Bandha Sarvangasana) can also help with alignment and proprioception.

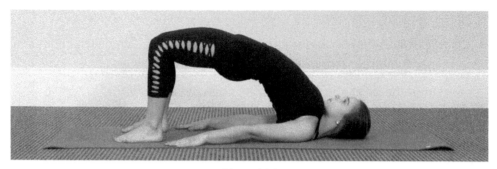

Figure 6.11

Precautions

Avoid if there is a neck injury. Do not let the knees push in towards each other or fall into each other due to hemiparesis. Do not move the head around during this pose—maintain a focus at a 45-degree angle.

Directions

1. Direct the client to start in supine position, bend the knees, and place the feet flat on the floor. They should bring the feet as close to the glutes as possible.

2. On an exhale, they should press the feet down into the floor and simultaneously push the hips off the floor. They should tighten the buttocks and maintain a parallel space between the thighs and knees, and push firmly onto the arms, which are extended under the body. Ask them to imagine the fingers reaching for the heels of each foot.

3. They should extend the hips until the thighs are approximately parallel to the floor. Direct them to use caution to keep the knees over the heels, and make sure that the knees stay parallel to each other.

4. They should lift the chin slightly, so that the back of the neck is on the ground and elongated. Ask them to imagine pushing the shoulder blades against the back and extending the shoulders away from the ears.

5. To release, roll the spine towards the ground slowly, one vertebra at a time if possible.

Modifications/Props

- To assist in raising the hips off the ground, a blanket or bolster can be placed under the sacrum (see Figure 6.12).

- A soft block placed under the sit bones makes this a restorative pose.

- A thick blanket under the shoulders can help to protect the neck.

- The pose can be accessed from a chair by sitting with the hips forward on the chair, slightly arching the back, and letting the elbows ground on the arm rests for support in the pose (see Figure 6.13).

- The wall can be used as support for a standing bridge (see Figure 6.14).

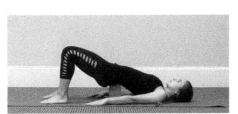

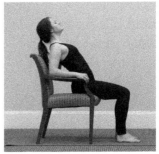

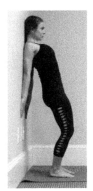

Figure 6.12

Figure 6.13

Figure 6.14

Cat Cow (Chakravakasana)

This pose is actually two poses that are frequently joined together because they flow well together. Cat pose (Marjariasana) (see Figure 6.15) and Cow pose (Bitilasana) (see Figure 6.16) combined make Cat Cow (Chakravakasana). Cat Cow (Chakravakasana) is a gentle stretch for the back, trunk, and neck, and is thought to reduce back pain. It creates space between the vertebrae. As these postures are in quadruped, the posture also helps with alignment and providing proprioceptive feedback to hemiparetic limbs.

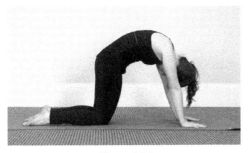

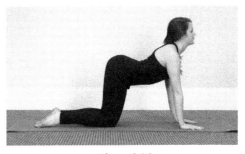

Figure 6.15

Figure 6.16

Precautions

Individuals with neck injuries should maintain a neutral position and not raise or curve the neck. Individuals with lower back problems should only perform Cow pose (Bitilasana) and then return the body to neutral instead of flowing to Cat pose (Marjariasana). Individuals with osteoporosis should move between neutral spine and Cow pose (Bitilasana), avoiding compression of the lumbar during deep forward folding. For clients with stroke who have a dense hemiparalysis, this posture may not be accessible or may only be completed with a lot of assistance from the therapist (or two therapists) and may require the use of a fold-down mat table instead of the floor. Quadruped is commonly included in post-stroke rehabilitation efforts and should be considered when using yoga as well.

Directions

1. Direct the client to start in Table Top (Goasana) (hands and knees on the floor), with the hands in front of the shoulders and the knees immediately below the hips. They should extend the fingers and press the palms into the floor.

2. Starting with Cat pose (Marjariasana), they should exhale and round the spine towards the ceiling. Tell them to keep the shoulders and knees in the same place and try not to move them. They should release the chin towards the chest, rounding gently.

3. They should inhale into Cow pose (Bitilasana), lifting the sitting bones and chest towards the ceiling. The back arches, the belly extends towards the floor, and the head lifts.

4. The flow between Cat (Marjariasana) and Cow (Bitilasana) poses continues by repeating Steps 2 and 3.

Modifications/Props

- A blanket under the knees can reduce strain on the knees.

- A blanket under the hands and wrists can reduce strain on the wrists. Cat Cow (Chakravakasana) can also be done with the forearms on the ground to reduce discomfort in the wrists.

- Having the forearms on a bolster helps to raise the ground closer to the individual, reducing strain on the shoulders and wrists (see Figures 6.17 and 6.18).

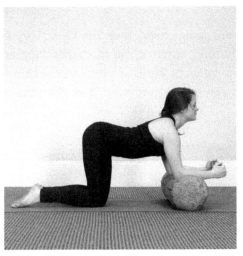

Figure 6.17

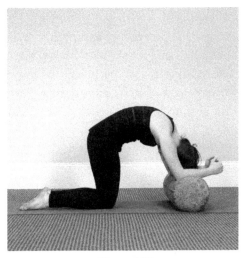

Figure 6.18

Chair Pose (Utkatasana)

Chair pose (Utkatasana) (see Figure 6.19) is a pose that requires a good deal of static and dynamic balance. Benefits of this pose include toning and strengthening the legs, ankles, and back, as well as stretching the chest and shoulders. Chair pose (Utkatasana) helps to activate the arches in the feet and stimulate the heart, diaphragm, and abdominal organs.

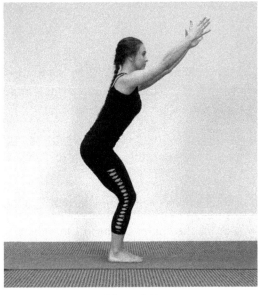

Figure 6.19

Precautions

Protect the knees by ensuring that they do not extend over the feet. This is contraindicated for people with low blood pressure, insomnia, and headaches. Proceed with caution if low back pain or lower extremity paralysis is present. Maintain a forward gaze if neck pain occurs. Perform the seated modification of the pose if dizziness occurs.

Directions

1. Direct the client to start in Mountain pose (Tadasana). Ask them to have the feet firmly planted on the floor with the feet touching. Ask them to imagine the four corners of each foot being rooted into the earth. The back should be straight with the head looking straight ahead.

2. They should inhale and extend the arms to approximately 45 degrees (diagonally) in front of the torso. The arms should be parallel, with the palms facing each other.

3. They should exhale and bend the knees. The full pose has the thighs parallel to the floor. Though that may not be accessible, they should move towards lowering the thighs while in this pose.

4. They should inhale, extend the arms, and firm the shoulder blades. Ask them to tuck the tailbone to elongate the spine.

5. They should exhale and release.

Modifications/Props

- This pose is easily modified to the wall by standing with the back a few inches away from the wall. The wall can provide a support for the tailbone, thus reducing threats to balance (see Figure 6.20).

- If the client has difficulty keeping the legs straight or together, adding a block between the knees and squeezing can help to bring attention to this area (see Figure 6.21).

- Use the back of the chair as needed for additional support.

- A rolled-up mat or blanket under the heels can reduce strain in the ankles.

- Arms in Prayer pose (Anjali Mudra) can reduce pain and discomfort in the back and upper body.

- Reduce the tilt forward to decrease the load on the muscles.

- The pose can be completed from a seated position by bringing the hips towards the front of the chair, leaning forward, and engaging the leg muscles as if one were about to stand up (see Figure 6.22).

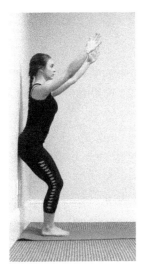
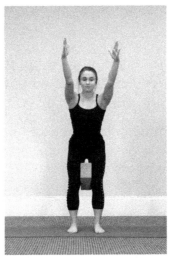
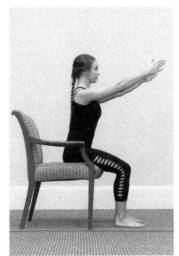

| *Figure 6.20* | *Figure 6.21* | *Figure 6.22* |

Child's Pose (Balasana)

Child's pose (Balasana) (see Figure 6.23) engages the parasympathetic nervous system and encourages the relaxation response. This pose also reduces strain in the neck, back, and hips, and calms the mind. Child's pose (Balasana) helps relieve anxiety, stress, and fatigue.

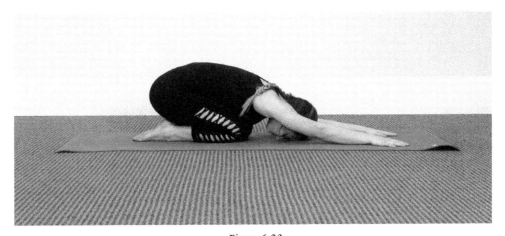

Figure 6.23

Precautions

If a knee injury is present, avoid this pose. This pose is contraindicated for people with diarrhea.

Directions

1. Ask the client to come into Table Top (Goasana). They should bring the toes together, bring the hips towards the heels, and separate the knees as wide as is comfortable—about the width of the hips.

2. They should relax the torso on top of the thighs and think about pushing the hips towards the heels. Ask them to imagine a long, stretched-out line between the top of the head and the bottom of the sacrum.

3. They should extend the arms and rest them on the floor for an active pose. For a more passive, resting pose, they could bring the arms along the side of the legs, maybe reaching the heels with the hands. Ask them to breathe into the spine and imagine the spine lengthening and widening. On exhalation, they should release deeper into the forward fold.

4. To release, ask them to raise the torso.

Modifications/Props

- A folded blanket or small bolster can be placed between the hamstrings and calves to reduce difficulty or pain with sitting on the heels.

- This pose can be done from a chair as part of a seated practice (see Figure 6.24).

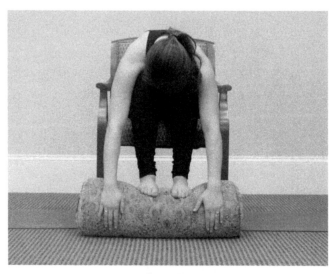

Figure 6.24

Cobra Pose (Bhujangasana)

Cobra pose (Bhujangasana) (see Figure 6.25) is done in a prone position and is designed to strengthen the spine and buttocks. This pose is also thought to stretch and stimulate the front of the body—including the chest, lungs, shoulders, and belly. Ancient texts indicate that this pose is helpful in increasing health and body temperature, as well as awakening the Kundalini energy. This pose helps improve proprioception and may be beneficial for hemiparesis.

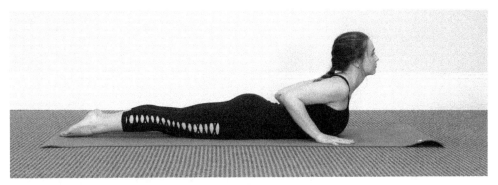

Figure 6.25

Precautions

Be careful in this pose if there is a back injury, carpal tunnel syndrome, or headache. Be cautious that the patient does not raise up too high on the straight arms or hyperextend the elbows.

Directions

1. Direct the client to lie prone on the floor. They should extend the legs back, with the toenails facing the floor.

2. They should bring the hands, palm down, under the shoulders. They should squeeze the elbows into the body.

3. They should press down on the feet and tighten the thighs and buttocks.

4. They should inhale, straighten the arms, and lift the chest. Ask them to keep the hips and legs touching the floor (don't straighten the arms so much that either come off the ground) and tuck the tailbone slightly.

5. They should raise the chest and sternum, and extend the shoulder blades down the back.

6. To release, they can exhale and lower the body carefully.

Modifications/Props

- This pose can be done at the wall or seated to reduce strain on the back (see Figures 6.26 and 6.27).

- To reduce strain on the lower back, the arms can be bent in an L shape with the forearms on the ground (this makes it Sphinx pose (Salamba Bhujangasana)).

- A blanket under the hips and pelvis helps to provide more space for the abdomen.

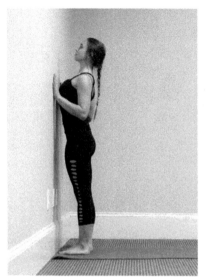

Figure 6.26

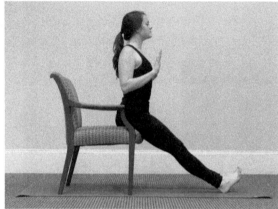

Figure 6.27

Corpse Pose (Savasana)

The Corpse pose (Savasana) (see Figure 6.28) is one of the most important postures because it allows the mind and body to rest after a physical practice. It allows the individual to soak in and integrate the benefits of the asanas that have preceded it. Corpse pose (Savasana) is thought to reduce blood pressure, calm the mind, and enhance relaxation throughout the body. It also reduces headache, fatigue, and insomnia. Typically, Corpse pose (Savasana) is completed at the end of the physical practice and is seen as a time for meditation and relaxation.

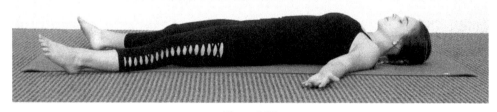

Figure 6.28

Precautions

Laying in supine position can strain the lower back, so placing a bolster underneath the knees helps to reduce that strain.

Directions

1. Direct the client to extend the body in a supine position.

2. The arms can be placed at the side or overhead, depending on individual preference. The palms should be placed face up. Ensure that the shoulder blades are both placed on the floor.

3. The legs should be extended to the width of the mat, with the feet turned out if that feels comfortable.

4. They should extend the neck and head towards the top of the mat.

5. Ask the client to soften the face, close the eyes if comfortable, relax the tongue, relax the cheeks, and soften the eyes.

6. A guideline for the length of time to spend in this pose is to practice Corpse pose (Savasana) for five minutes for every 30 minutes of physical practice.

7. To release, ask them to bring the attention back to the room. They should roll onto the right side and then press the body up, with the head coming up last.

8. They can apply an eye pillow to enhance relaxation. Read about application of the eye pillow and other benefits in Chapter 5.

Modifications/Props

- Raise the head by putting a rolled-up blanket under the neck and/or head (see Figure 6.29).

- Recline on a bolster.

- Place a bolster under the knees to reduce strain on the lower back.

- The knees can also stay bent, and a strap can bind the thighs.

- Sandbags can be placed on the different limbs or the pelvic area to provide a feeling of grounding.

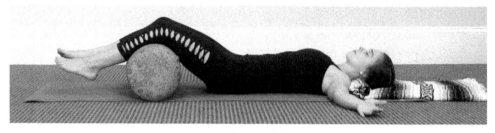

Figure 6.29

Crescent Lunge, High or Low (Anjeneyasana)

Crescent Lunge (Anjeneyasana) (see Figure 6.30) can be done in a knee-down (low) or knee-raised (high) position. Crescent Lunge (Anjeneyasana) is thought to open the hips and release tension housed in the hips. It also provides stretching for the quadriceps, groin, and hamstrings. Crescent Lunge (Anjeneyasana) is thought to increase mental clarity and focus. Crescent Lunge (Anjeneyasana) may stretch the hip flexors, which are often very tight in clients with stroke.

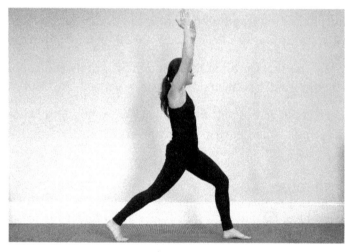

Figure 6.30

Precautions

This pose is contraindicated for individuals with high blood pressure and heart problems. Ensure that the back is not arched too much when the torso is raised.

Directions

1. Direct the client to begin in Downward Facing Dog (Adho Mukha Svanasana).

2. They should exhale and bring the right foot between the hands.

3. They should drop the left knee to the mat (gently) for Low Crescent Lunge (Anjeneyasana), or keep the knee raised and the left leg strong for High Crescent Lunge (Anjeneyasana).

4. They should inhale, bring the torso upright, and raise the arms overhead.

5. They should reach back with the left heel to increase the extension of the leg, and bring the shoulders together and down the back. The gaze can be forward or towards the extended hands.

6. They should exhale with the hands coming down to the mat and the right foot meeting the left at the back of the mat in Downward Facing Dog (Adho Mukha Svanasana) for High Crescent Lunge (Anjeneyasana) or Child's pose (Balasana) for Low Crescent Lunge (Anjeneyasana).

7. They should repeat with the left foot forward.

Modifications/Props

- If doing a seated practice, this pose is accessible from a seated position (see Figure 6.31).

- If this is uncomfortable for the knee on the ground in Low Crescent Lunge (Anjeneyasana), the mat can be folded up under the knee or a blanket or other support can be placed under the knee (see Figure 6.32).

- To help with balance, the toes of the front foot could be close to the wall. Reach the arms up and rest the fingers on the wall (see Figure 6.33).

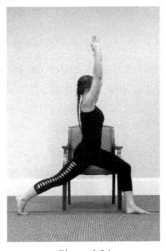 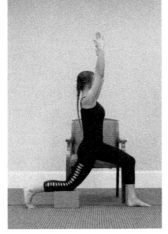 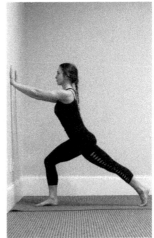

Figure 6.31   *Figure 6.32*   *Figure 6.33*

Downward Facing Dog (Adho Mukha Svanasana)

Downward Facing Dog (Adho Mukha Svanasana) (see Figure 6.34) is a pose that is used in most yoga classes. It has a number of benefits, including: elongating and decompressing the spine; stretching the hamstrings, shoulders, calves, arches of the feet, and the hands; strengthening the arms and legs; enhancing oxygen flow to the brain; calming the mind; improving digestion; helping to relieve stress; and providing energy for the body and mind.

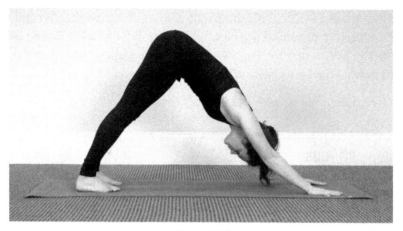

Figure 6.34

Precautions

This pose has the head below the heart, so modify or avoid it if the blood pressure is high and in the acute phases after stroke.

Directions

1. Direct the client to start in Table Top (Goasana) (hands and knees on the floor). The hands should be in front of the shoulders and the knees should be immediately below the hips. They should extend the fingers and press the palms into the floor, and bring the toes under the feet.

2. On an exhale, they should pull the knees away from the floor and extend the tailbone towards the ceiling. The knees can stay bent if needed, based on hamstring flexibility. The goal of the posture is to bring the heels towards the ground with the legs straight.

3. Focusing on the arms, they should externally rotate the triceps and push the base of the index fingers into the floor. Ask them to feel the shoulder blades widen across the back and towards the feet. They should not let the head hang. Direct the client to maintain the focus of the eyes (drishti) between the hands.

Modifications/Props

- This asana can be difficult for people with tight hamstrings. Use blocks under each hand to bring the floor closer to the individual.

- The head can be propped on blocks or bolsters so that it does not hang.

- At the wall, stand with the arms extended and the hands touching the wall so that the arms are parallel to each other. Activate the arms as described in Step 3 of the directions above (see Figures 6.35 and 6.36).

- Stand with the arms extended, touching the top of a chair. The body is in an L shape.

- Place a blanket under the wrists if the hands or wrists hurt.

- This could be done as part of a seated practice (see Figure 6.37).

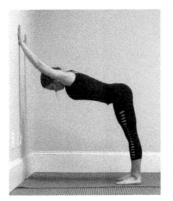
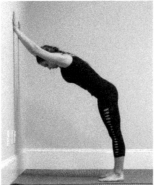
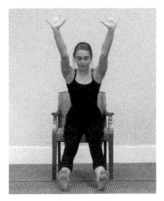

| *Figure 6.35* | *Figure 6.36* | *Figure 6.37* |

Eagle (Garudasana)—Arms Only

The full Eagle (Garudasana) posture requires complex balance skills. However, the arm posture can be used alone (see Figure 6.38), which stretches the shoulders and upper back. This posture also promotes enhanced concentration. For people who are post-stroke, this posture may help to stretch the shoulders, which may be tighter due to spasticity or increased tone in the upper body.

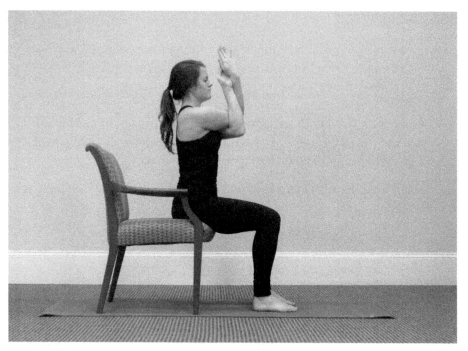

Figure 6.38

Precautions

Use caution with anyone with an arm or shoulder injury, such as a post-stroke subluxed shoulder.

Directions

1. Direct the client to stand in Mountain pose (Tadasana).

2. They should extend the arms out to the left and right.

3. They should inhale, bringing the right arm under the left.

4. When the elbows meet, they should bring the right arm upright so that the fingers are pointed to the ceiling.

5. They should flex the left arm and bring the palms/hands to touch.

6. They should raise the arms so that elbows are at shoulder height. Ask them to expand the scapulas across the back and press the hands into each other.

7. They should release the arms and repeat on the other side.

Modifications/Props

- This is a difficult arm posture. To make this more accessible, cross the right arm over the left and move towards having the elbows stacked on top of each other and grasping the shoulder or upper arm of the opposite arm (see Figure 6.39).

- Another modification is to bring the hands to Prayer pose (Anjali Mudra) and move the forearms and elbows together to make one straight line from the elbow to fingertips (see Figure 6.40).

- This pose could be done seated or with the back to the wall for additional support.

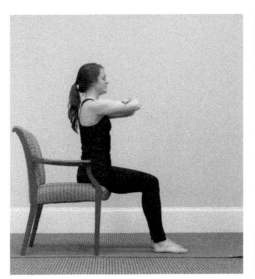

Figure 6.39

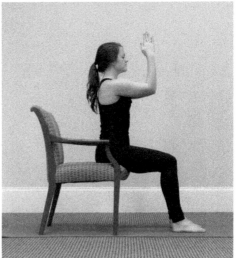

Figure 6.40

Easy Pose (Sukhasana)

Easy pose (Sukhasana) (see Figure 6.41) is one that most people are accustomed to doing—it is a typical crossed-leg position that typically occurs sitting on the floor. While it seems easy, it can be difficult for people with tight quadriceps or hemiparesis. Easy pose (Sukhasana) is a hip opener that produces feelings of calm and decreases anxiety. Sitting in Easy pose (Sukhasana) with a straight back can strengthen the back and improve posture.

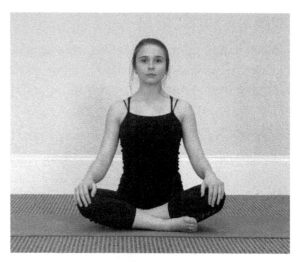

Figure 6.41

Precautions

None noted.

Directions

1. Direct the client to start in a seated position and extend the legs in front of the body in Staff pose (Rekha).

2. They should cross the shins, and place each foot under the opposite knee, drawing the feet towards the body.

3. The pelvis should be in a neutral position.

4. They should lengthen the spine and extend the head towards the ceiling.

5. The hands can rest in the lap or on the knees.

Modifications/Props

• Place blocks under each knee if the knees are high off the ground (see Figure 6.42).

• Place a folded blanket under the hips for support and a more comfortable seat (see Figure 6.43).

• This can be modified for a seated chair practice (see Figure 6.44).

• Sit with the back near the wall and put a yoga block between the wall and the back to provide support for sitting (see Figure 6.45).

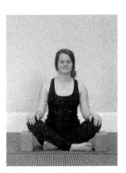
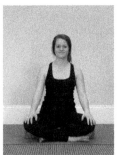
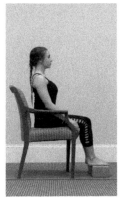
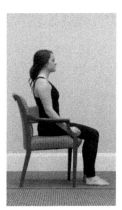

| Figure 6.42 | Figure 6.43 | Figure 6.44 | Figure 6.45 |

Extended Side Angle (Utthita Parsvakonasana)

Extended Side Angle (Utthita Parsvakonasana) (see Figure 6.46) is a standing pose that requires strong balance. It is thought to stretch the side body, waist, shoulders, and groin, as well as to stretch and strengthen the lower extremities. Extended Side Angle (Utthita Parsvakonasana) is also thought to stimulate the abdominal organs and enhance stamina.

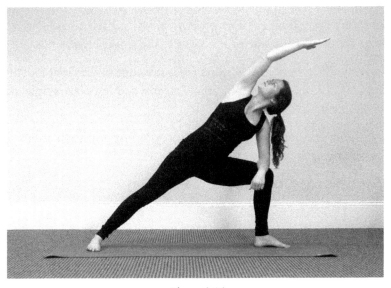

Figure 6.46

Precautions

Extended Side Angle (Utthita Parsvakonasana) is contraindicated for people with headaches, high or low blood pressure, and insomnia. Individuals with neck issues should maintain a neutral neck and not look up towards the arm that is overhead.

Directions

1. Direct the client to move into Warrior II (Virabhadrasana II):

    i. Ask them to start in Mountain pose (Tadasana). They should inhale, exhale, and extend the right foot back in a high lunge position, modifying the right foot to extend to the right at a 90-degree angle. The left foot should be pointing straight ahead, with the left knee bent and the left foot directly under the left knee.

    ii. They should rotate the hips and pelvis so they are parallel with the long side of the yoga mat.

    iii. They should extend the arms, so that the left arm is over the left bent knee, and the right arm is over the right straight leg. Ask them to bring the gaze over the middle finger of the left hand, stretch the arms away from each other, and energetically pull the shoulder blades apart from each other.

2. They should exhale and bring the left arm to rest above the left knee. Ask them to turn the chest towards the ceiling.

3. They should bring the right arm overhead, with the fingers extended towards the ceiling. The right palm should be facing the long side of the mat overhead.

4. Ask them to turn the head to look towards the right arm and release the shoulders away from the ears on both sides. Suggest they focus on creating length along the left side of the torso as the right side extends.

5. They should intentionally ground the outer edge of the right foot on the floor and extend through the right arm. The arm and leg on the right side should be one long line.

6. To release, they can bend the front knee slightly and push against it, pulling the torso into the upright position.

7. They should repeat on the other side.

Modifications/Props

- Step on a sandbag or rolled-up mat to help maintain the back foot on the ground.

- The arms may feel more stable in Prayer pose (Anjali Mudra).

- A chair may help to provide stability. Place it parallel with the long side of the mat.

- This pose is easily adapted to being done in a seated position (see Figure 6.47).

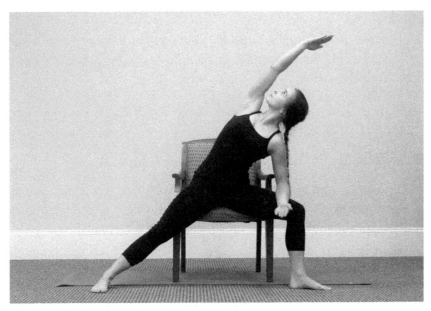

Figure 6.47

Five Pointed Star or Star Pose (Utthita Tadasana)

Five Pointed Star pose (Utthita Tadasana) (see Figure 6.48) elongates and stretches the body in all directions simultaneously. This asana brings the spine into proper alignment and strengthens the lower body. It is thought to improve circulation and respiration, as well as to reduce stress and improve concentration.

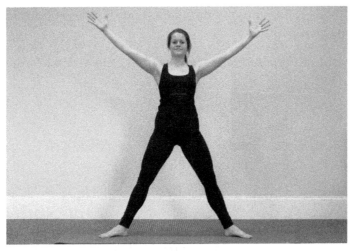

Figure 6.48

Precautions

Five Pointed Star pose (Utthita Tadasana) is a standing posture; thus if there are balance concerns, additional attention should be taken by following one of the modifications offered below.

Directions

1. Direct the client to begin in Mountain pose (Tadasana).

2. Ask them to turn to the right, facing the long side of the mat, and step the legs wide apart. They should extend the toes out slightly (no more than 45 degrees), pointing towards the corners of the mat.

3. They should extend both arms at shoulder height with the thumbs up and fingers extended. The feet should be close to underneath each wrist.

4. They should expand the arms and legs energetically and imagine sending energy out through the palms of each hand and the ball of each foot. Direct them to use caution to not hyperextend through the arms or legs.

5. They should engage the thighs by activating the quadriceps.

6. They should tuck the tailbone slightly without rounding the lower back.

7. They should extend the torso and reach the crown of the head towards the ceiling.

8. They should broaden across the front of the chest, particularly along the collarbones, and bring the shoulder blades together but not squeeze them. Tell them to maintain straight and firm arms.

9. They should release the arms and return them to Mountain pose (Tadasana).

Modifications/Props

- This asana can be done with the back against the wall or with one hand against the wall for stability (see Figure 6.49).

- Arms can be in Prayer pose (Anjali Mudra) at the front of the chest.

- This pose can be done from a chair as part of a seated practice (see Figure 6.50).

- This pose inherently includes contralateral movement. If modified to a chair or wall, try to maintain some contralateral movement in the pose.

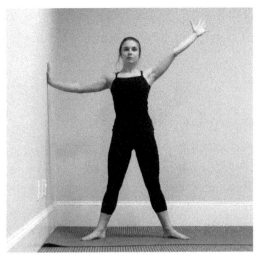

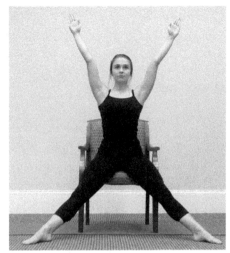

Figure 6.49   *Figure 6.50*

Goddess or Fierce Angle Pose (Utkata Konasana)

Goddess pose (Utkata Konasana) (see Figure 6.51) is a standing pose that is similar in many ways to Five Pointed Star pose (Utthita Tadasana). Goddess pose (Utkata Konasana) is thought to strengthen the calves, quadriceps, inner thighs, and core, as well as the shoulders, arms, and upper back. The pose also stretches the muscles of the hips, groin, and chest, which may be tighter following a stroke.

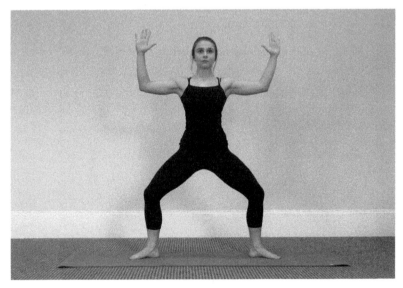

Figure 6.51

Precautions

The knees should point in the same direction as the toes to help protect the knees.

Directions

1. Direct the client to begin in Mountain pose (Tadasana).

2. Ask them to turn right to face the long side of the mat and step the legs wide apart. They should extend the toes out to approximately 45 degrees, pointing towards the corners of the mat, and tuck the tailbone slightly without rounding the back.

3. They should extend both arms at shoulder height with the thumbs up and fingers extended. The feet should be close to underneath each wrist.

4. They should expand the arms and legs energetically; ask them to imagine sending energy out through the palms of each hand and the ball of each foot. They should use caution to not hyperextend through the arms or legs.

5. They should engage the thighs by engaging the quadriceps.

6. They should extend the torso and reach the crown of the head towards the ceiling.

7. They should broaden across the front of the chest, particularly along the collarbones.

8. They should bring the shoulder blades together, but not squeeze them, and maintain straight and firm arms.

9. They should bend at the knees and bring the thighs parallel to the ground, and ensure that the knees remain directly over the ankles. From extended arms, they can turn the palms up and bring the elbows into the sides with the palms up. This results in a squatting-type position with the arms and legs bent simultaneously.

10. They should release the arms and return to Mountain pose (Tadasana).

Modifications/Props

- This asana can be done with the back to the wall for stability.

- This asana can be done from a seated position (see Figure 6.52).

- The arms can be in Prayer pose (Anjali Mudra) at the front of the chest.

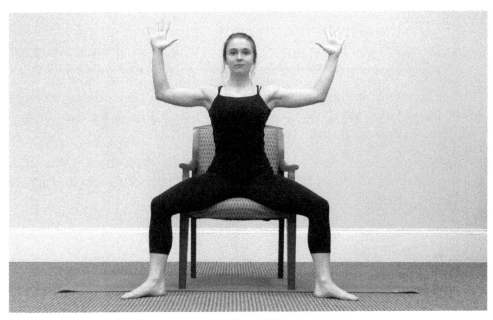

Figure 6.52

Happy Baby or Dead Bug Pose (Ananda Balasana)

Happy Baby pose (Ananda Balasana) (see Figure 6.53) is a supine posture that provides a moment of relaxation with a stretch to the low back and hips. Happy Baby pose (Ananda Balasana) gently stretches the inner thigh and groin muscles and provides stimulation for the spine. It also helps to calm the mind and reduce stress.

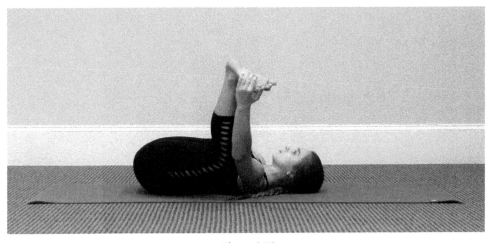

Figure 6.53

Precautions

Proceed with caution or avoid for those with back or groin injuries.

Directions

1. Direct the client to start in a supine position. They should inhale, exhale, and bring the knees into 90 degrees. The knees should be near the belly.

2. They should inhale, reach for the pinky side of the feet or the big toes, and increase the width of the knees so that they are wider than the torso and pull the knees into the chest.

3. The feet should be flexed directly above the knee so the shins are perpendicular to the floor. They should flex the heels and push the feet against the hands to feel resistance.

Modifications/Props

*   A strap or gait belt can be used to extend the reach—place the strap or belt around the soles of the feet and hold each end firmly.

*   This can be done as a Half Happy Baby pose (Ardha Ananda Balasana), by holding one foot at a time.

*   This can be done from a seated position (see Figure 6.54).

*   If the feet are not accessible, the thighs or knees can be held instead.

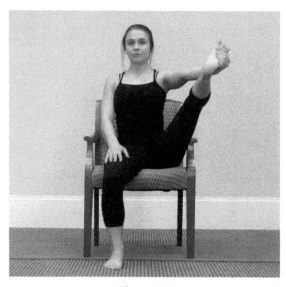

Figure 6.54

Knees to Chest or Supine Knees to Chest Pose (Apanasana)

This pose (see Figure 6.55) provides relief from digestive issues, including indigestion, bloating, flatulence, and acidity.

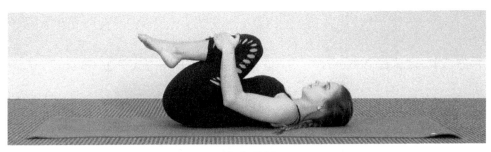

Figure 6.55

Precautions

Avoid if a knee, hip, or spinal injury is present. If a neck injury is present, do not lift the head in this asana.

Directions

1. Direct the client to lie prone, with the legs and arms extended.

2. They should inhale, exhale, and draw both knees to the chest. If possible, they can wrap the forearms around the shins and clasp each elbow with the opposite hand.

3. They should ensure that the back maintains contact with the mat, release their shoulder blades away from the ears, and broaden the chest.

4. They should pull the tailbone towards the mat, and feel the spine lengthen even more.

5. If it feels good, they can slowly rock the back from front to back or side to side for a gentle spinal massage.

6. They should tuck the chin slightly.

7. Ask them to focus on breathing evenly.

8. They should exhale, release, and extend both legs along the floor and rest.

Modifications/Props

- If it is difficult to clasp both hands around the legs:
  - each arm can be held behind the knee on the same side of the body
  - use a gait belt or yoga strap to elongate the reach and wrap it around the soles of both feet to pull the knees in towards the body. A gait belt or yoga strap used in this manner can also engage the affected side.

- For neck discomfort or difficulty engaging the head, place a blanket under the head.

- This can be done from a seated position in a chair (see Figure 6.56).

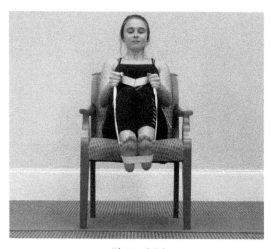

Figure 6.56

Lion's Pose (Simhasana)

Lion's pose (Simhasana) (see Figure 6.57) is a posture that has a lot of benefits but can be done in a variety of settings. This posture is primarily one of the face, but also involves breath and coordination, and often makes people laugh. This pose is thought to reduce tension and improve circulation in the facial muscles as well as helping to keep the eyes healthy. This pose also firms the platysma—a muscle on the front of the neck—as well as treating bad breath. Lion's pose (Simhasana) may positively impact some of the muscles that are associated with dysarthria.

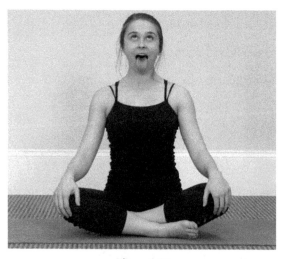

Figure 6.57

Precautions

None noted.

Directions

1. Direct the client to start by kneeling on the floor with the knees shoulder width apart.

2. They should lift the chest towards the ceiling.

3. They should place the hands with wide palms and outstretched fingers on each knee.

4. They should inhale deeply through the nose.

5. Ask them to make the following movements simultaneously.

    i.   Open the mouth as wide as possible.

    ii.   Extend the tongue and curl the tip of the tongue towards the chin.

    iii. Open the eyes and look up towards the eyebrows.

    iv.   Contract the muscles at the front of the throat.

    v.   Extend the fingers, like a lion's claws.

6. They should hold the position and exhale slowly through the mouth, and make a "haaaaa" sound with the exhale.

7. They should roar like a lion.

8. They should retract the tongue and relax the face.

9. Ask them to repeat several times.

Modifications/Props

*   This posture can easily be modified for a seated or standing position (see Figure 6.58), as included in the sample practices in Chapter 12.

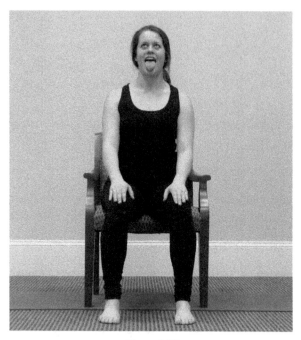

Figure 6.58

Locust Pose (Salabhasana)

Locust pose (Salabhasana) (see Figure 6.59) is a prone position that strengthens the back of the body, including the arms and legs. It also stimulates the belly, relieves stress, and stretches the shoulders and chest, as well as the belly and thighs. This pose helps improve proprioception and may be beneficial for hemiparesis.

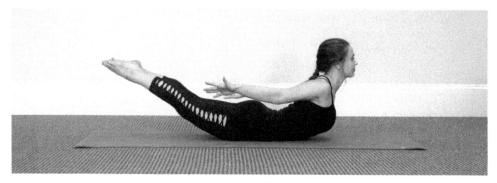

Figure 6.59

Precautions

Use caution with individuals with back injuries or headache. Patients with neck injuries should maintain a neutral neck, keeping the gaze at the floor, or be supported by a folded blanket.

Directions

1. Direct the client to lie prone on the mat and bring the arms alongside the body, with the palms facing up. The forehead rests on the floor.

2. They should firm the buttocks, exhale, and lift the head, chest, and torso away from the mat. They should extend through the legs and pull the feet up while the upper body is elevated off the mat. The belly and hips should be pressing into the floor. They should tuck the tailbone slightly to increase support for and pressure on the buttocks and pelvis.

3. Ask them to extend actively through the feet and arms. The torso and head should lift towards the ceiling without crunching the lower back. They should press the shoulder blades firmly down the back.

4. The gaze should be forward or slightly up. Ask them to exhale and release.

Modifications/Props

- A rolled-up blanket or small bolster under the hip bones will help to provide elevation and space for Locust pose (Salabhasana).

- A rolled-up blanket or small bolster under the feet may provide support to help raise the legs.

- This posture can be split into legs only, upper body only, or even one leg at a time.

- From a seated chair position, this asana can be completed by leaning forward, bringing the arms behind, and drawing the shoulder blades together (see Figure 6.60).

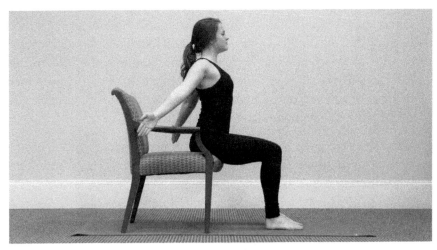

Figure 6.60

Mountain Pose (Tadasana)

Mountain pose (Tadasana) (see Figure 6.61) is the foundation for most standing asanas. This asana is thought to reduce flat feet and improve posture, strengthen the lower body, and firm the belly and buttocks.

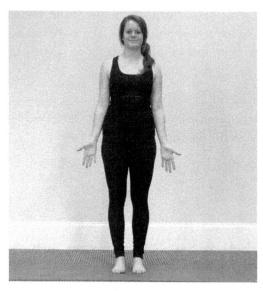

Figure 6.61

Precautions

As with all standing postures, use caution with someone with low blood pressure. This asana may be contraindicated for individuals with headache and insomnia.

Directions

1. Direct the client to stand upright and bring the big toes together, with the heels of the feet slightly apart. They should lift all ten toes and spread them as wide as possible. While energetically pushing into the balls of the feet, they should lower the toes. Ask them to imagine the four corners of each foot being anchored into the ground (under the base of the big toe, under the base of the pinky toe, and both lateral sides of the heel).

2. They should engage the core and tuck the tailbone slightly. They should firm the quadriceps and lift the knees, allowing the arches of both feet to lift while the feet remain planted.

3. They should bring the shoulders towards the ears, release the shoulders down the back, and broaden. They should allow the arms to be at the sides, with the palms facing forward.

4. The head should be aligned over the neck and the middle of the pelvis. They should keep the chin parallel to the floor, and lift the chest and sternum towards the ceiling while maintaining a straight back.

Modifications/Props

- Doing Mountain pose (Tadasana) against a wall will provide feedback about the length and straightness of the spine.

- Increasing the base of support increases balance.

- Use the back of a chair to provide additional support.

- This pose can be modified to a seated position (see Figure 6.62).

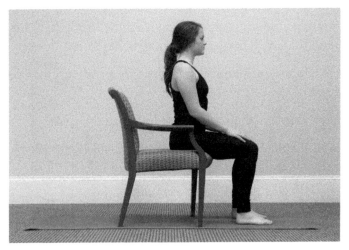

Figure 6.62

Plank (Kumbhakasana)

Plank (Kumbhakasana) (see Figure 6.63) is done in a prone position. It is thought to strengthen the arms, wrists, and spine and tone the belly.

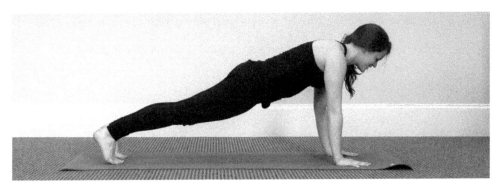

Figure 6.63

Precautions

This is contraindicated for people with carpal tunnel syndrome, but the forearm modification (noted below) may make this pose accessible for someone with carpal tunnel syndrome. Clients with dense hemiplegia may need to use a modified version as outlined below.

Directions

1. There are several ways to start this pose, but it is likely most accessible if starting in a prone position on the floor.

2. Direct the client to bend the knees and place the hands on the floor under the shoulders. They should push to straighten the arms and raise the torso off the ground. The upper body should be in a straight line.

3. If it's available to the client, they can plant the toes and lift the knees off the ground so the whole body is in a straight line.

4. They should externally rotate the upper arms and grip the floor firmly with the fingers.

5. They should spread the shoulder blades across the spine.

6. The head should be in line with the body and should not be hanging, but with the gaze at the floor.

7. The thighs should also be externally rotating, and the legs should be pressing towards the heels.

Modifications/Props

- This pose can easily be modified to the wall, by standing and pushing on the wall instead of moving into a prone position (see Figure 6.64).

- The hands and fingers can be pressed against the corner of a wall/floor and the crown of the head pressed into the wall to experience stability from the wall.

- Instead of extending arms, the individual can rest on the forearms.

- This could also be completed from a seated position (see Figure 6.65).

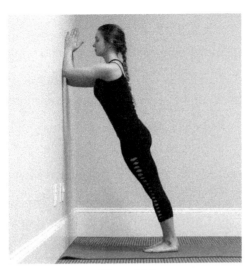

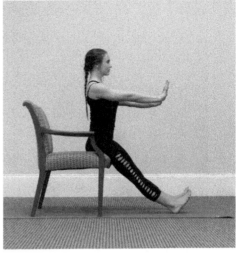

Figure 6.64   *Figure 6.65*

Reclining Spinal Twist or Master Revolved Abdomen Pose (Jathara Parivartanasana)

This asana (see Figure 6.66) is a supine-position, reclining Spinal Twist (Jathara Parivartanasana), which helps to enhance flexibility and strength in the belly and improves circulation throughout the belly.

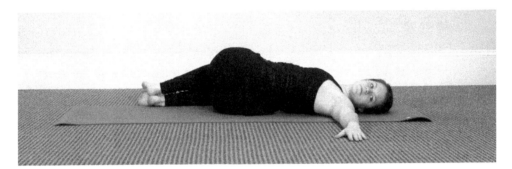

Figure 6.66

Precautions

Ensure that the knees do not shift below the pelvis. For people with neck issues, make sure the neck is not twisted when the body twists. The head and neck can point in the same direction as the knees to eliminate discomfort or concern.

Directions

1. Direct the client to start in supine extension (lying flat on the back) and bring the knees into the chest.

2. They should do several repetitions of breathing—inhalation and exhalation.

3. They should extend each arm straight to the left and right, with the palms up and in line with the shoulders.

4. They should exhale and drop the knees to the right towards the right elbow.

5. They should use the pressure between the extended left arm and the ground to counterbalance the twist. Try to keep the left shoulder blade on the floor.

6. They should inhale and lengthen the torso and then exhale and increase the twist.

7. They should repeat on the left side.

Modifications/Props

• If bringing both the knees in simultaneously is too intense, this pose can be done as a half reclining Spinal Twist (Jathara Parivartanasana), by bringing one knee over at a time. If that is too intense, a bolster can be placed under the revolved knee for support (see Figure 6.67).

• A block can be placed in between the knees to reduce strain if both knees are revolved.

• This posture can be done when reclining on a bolster that is placed perpendicular to the torso so that the head and torso are above the knees.

• During a seated practice, a Spinal Twist (Jathara Parivartanasana) can be done by beginning in Mountain pose (Tadasana) and rotating the torso (see Figure 6.68).

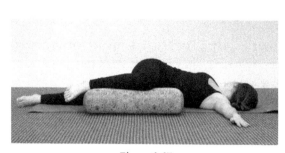

Figure 6.67

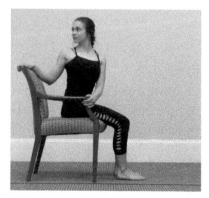

Figure 6.68

Seated Forward Fold (Paschimottanasana)

This posture (see Figure 6.69) is thought to reduce pain such as headaches, calm the mind, and relieve anxiety and depression. Seated Forward Fold (Paschimottanasana) is also thought to stimulate the organs of the liver, kidneys, ovaries, and uterus, as well as to improve digestion. This posture stretches the back, spine, shoulders, and hamstrings.

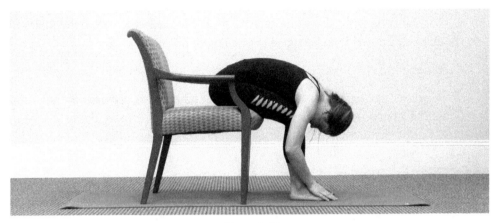

Figure 6.69

Precautions

It is important to not force the forward fold, which could result in tearing a hamstring or the lower back muscles. This pose is contraindicated for people with diarrhea and back injuries.

Directions

1. Direct the client to sit on the floor or a chair with the legs extended, flex the feet, and press through the heels.

2. They should move the flesh under the sit bones by putting the weight onto one buttock, and then the other, and moving the flesh away.

3. They should inhale, raise the arms, contract the belly, and lean forward from the hips. Ask them to try to keep the back straight and grasp the toes or, if that is not available or not comfortable, use a strap to reach towards the toes.

4. With each inhale, they should raise the chest and lengthen; with each exhale, they should release more into the fold.

5. To release the fold, they should lift the chest, tuck the tailbone, and come into an upright position.

Modifications/Props

- Sitting on a blanket, particularly with the blanket under the sit bones, can reduce some strain. Raising this seat further, such as by using blocks as well, can enhance the stretch and reduce the strain.

- A strap or gait belt can be very helpful in moving into this pose.

- For someone with very tight hamstrings, the legs can be bent at the knees to make this pose more manageable (see Figure 6.70).

- If done in a chair, blocks can be placed under the feet to help the knees bend.

- A bolster can be placed between the legs and belly to decrease the intensity of the stretch in the spine (see Figure 6.71).

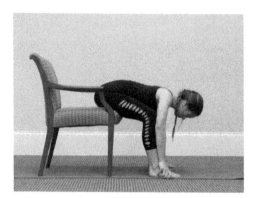

Figure 6.70

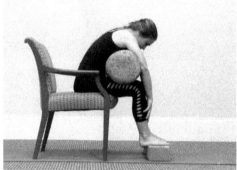

Figure 6.71

Shooting Star Pose (Eka Pada Utthita Tadasana)

This pose (see Figure 6.72) is very similar to Five Pointed Star pose (Utthita Tadasana). It is a one-legged standing pose that challenges balance. It has the same benefits as Five Pointed Star pose (Utthita Tadasana): it elongates and stretches the body in all directions simultaneously. This asana brings the spine into proper alignment and strengthens the lower body. It is also thought to improve circulation and respiration, as well as to reduce stress and improve concentration.

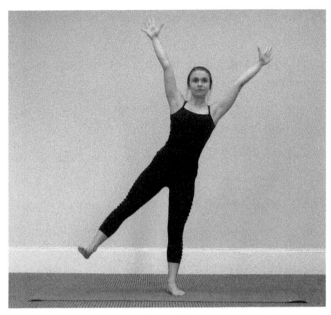

Figure 6.72

Precautions

This is a standing posture on one leg; thus if there are balance concerns, additional attention should be given.

Directions

1. Direct the client to begin in Five Pointed Star pose (Utthita Tadasana):

   i. They should start in Mountain pose (Tadasana).

   ii. Ask them to turn to the right, facing the long side of the mat, and step the legs wide apart. They should extend the toes out slightly (no more than 45 degrees), pointing towards the corners of the mat.

   iii. They should extend both arms at shoulder height with the thumbs up and fingers extended. The feet should be close to underneath each wrist.

   iv. They should expand the arms and legs energetically; ask them to imagine sending energy out through the palms of each hand and the ball of each foot. They should use caution to not hyperextend through the arms or legs.

   v. They should engage the thighs by activating the quadriceps.

   vi. They should tuck the tailbone slightly without rounding the lower back.

vii. They should extend the torso and reach the crown of the head towards the ceiling.

viii. They should broaden across the front of the chest, particularly along the collarbones.

ix. They should bring the shoulder blades together, but not squeeze them, and maintain straight and firm arms.

2. They should transfer the weight to the right leg, and lift the left leg off the ground.

3. They should release the arms and return to Mountain pose (Tadasana).

4. Ask them to repeat on the right side.

Modifications/Props

- This asana can be done by leaning one arm against the wall for stability (see Figure 6.73).

- The arms can be in Prayer pose (Anjali Mudra) at the front of the chest.

- Use the back of the chair for additional support (see Figure 6.74).

- The posture can be done from a seated position by starting from Mountain pose (Tadasana), extending the arms, and lifting and extending one leg (see Figure 6.75). This is a contralateral exercise if the opposite arm is extended as well.

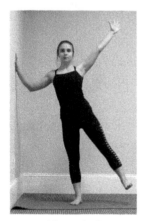
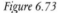

Figure 6.73

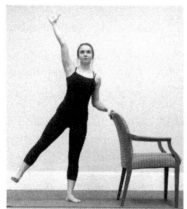

Figure 6.74

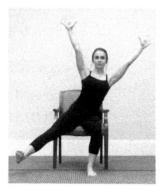

Figure 6.75

Sphinx Pose (Salamba Bhujangasana)

Sphinx pose (Salamba Bhujangasana) (see Figure 6.76) is done in prone position, with the forearms under the shoulders. This pose offers the same benefits as Cobra pose (Bhujangasana), without the strain on the wrists. It is thought to stretch and stimulate the front of the body, including the chest, lungs, shoulders, and belly. Ancient texts indicate that this pose is helpful in increasing health and body temperature, as well as awakening the Kundalini energy. This pose helps improve proprioception and may be beneficial for hemiparesis.

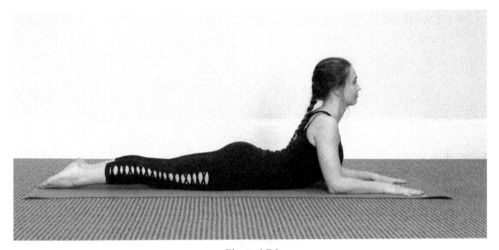

Figure 6.76

Precautions

Be careful in this pose if there is a back injury, carpal tunnel syndrome, or headache. Though the arms should not be straight in the pose, be cautious during transitions that the client does not raise up too high on straight arms or hyperextend the elbows.

Directions

1. Direct the client to lie prone on the floor and extend the legs back, with the toenails facing the floor.

2. They should lift the head and place the forearms on the floor, parallel to each other. They should lift the torso enough to bring the forearms under the torso and squeeze the elbows into the body.

3. They should press down on the feet and tighten the thighs and buttocks.

4. They should inhale and lift the head and chest. Ask them to keep the hip bones and legs touching the floor (and not to straighten the arms so much that either come off the ground), and tuck the tailbone slightly.

5. They should raise the chest and sternum. Extend the shoulder blades down the back.

6. To release, they can exhale and lower the body carefully.

Modifications/Props

- A blanket under the hips and pelvis helps to provide more space for the abdomen.

- For clients with dense hemiplegia, this pose may be completed at the wall to reduce the weight bearing required by the arms (see Figure 6.77).

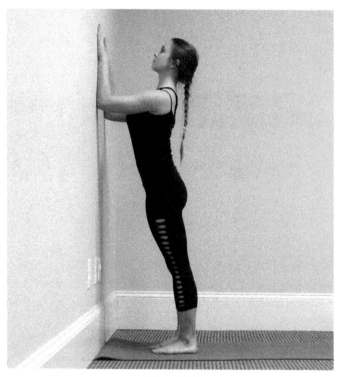

Figure 6.77

Standing Forward Fold (Uttanasana)

Forward folds (see Figures 6.78 and 6.79) are nice transitions and offer an opportunity to rest, but they should be used carefully with people with stroke because the head is below the heart, so please note the Half Forward Fold (Ardha Uttanasana) modification offered below. Forward folds are known to calm the brain and stretch the back of the legs (including the hamstrings and calves), while strengthening the front of the leg (including the thighs and knees). Forward folds may also reduce fatigue and anxiety and reduce headaches.

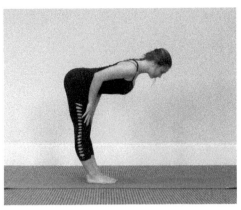

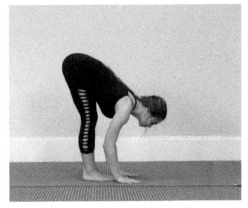

Figure 6.78   *Figure 6.79*

Precautions

This may challenge the balance of an individual with stroke. Use caution.

Directions

1. Direct the client to start in Mountain pose (Tadasana). They should have the legs together and feet anchored into the ground. They should place the hands on the hips and inhale.

2. They should bend the knees slightly, exhale, and bend forward, bending from the hips, not the waist. They should bend as far forward as possible, and place the hands where they land—on the knees, shins, feet, or floor. They should relax the head. Ask them to imagine lifting the tailbone to the ceiling.

3. To release, they can bend the knees, bring the hands to the hips, and raise the torso as one unit. They should tuck the tailbone and come up to an upright position.

Modifications/Props

- Half Forward Fold (Ardha Uttanasana) is a better choice for a person with acute stroke, high blood pressure, or back pain. This can be done at the wall, with the arms parallel to the floor and hands on the wall at waist height (see Figure 6.80).

- Place a rolled-up mat or sandbag under the heels (but not the entire foot) to reduce some strain on the lower back.

- Complete the forward fold while seated in a chair (see Figure 6.69), as included in the sample practices in Chapter 12.

- If completed while seated, a bolster may be used to reduce the strain in the back and hamstrings (see Figure 6.71).

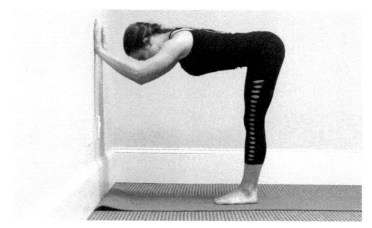

Figure 6.80

Supine Pigeon, Figure 4, or Threading the Needle (Supta Eka Pada Rajakapotasana)

This supine version of Pigeon (see Figure 6.81) brings the benefits of this posture to those who prefer not, or who are not able, to extend into full Pigeon. This pose increases the flexibility of the hips and lengthens the hamstrings and hip flexors.

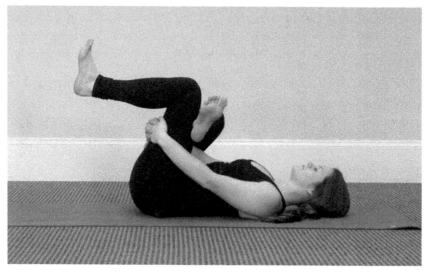

Figure 6.81

Precautions

Ensure that both hips stay placed on the floor.

Directions

1. Direct the client to begin in a supine position. They should bend the knees so that the feet are resting on the floor.

2. They should cross the right ankle at the left knee so that the ankle is on the femur side of the knee.

3. They should extend the right arm through the space between the bent right leg and the left leg. They should grasp the left hand with the right hand behind the left thigh.

4. They should relax the head and back of the neck on the floor.

5. They should pull the arms and legs in towards the chest, gently, just until a stretch is felt.

6. They should release the arms and legs and repeat on the other side.

Modifications/Props

- A strap or gait belt can be used to extend the reach of the hands.

- Instead of reaching through the legs, the legs can be pulled in towards the chest without use of the arms.

- A bolster placed at the buttocks may help an individual stay in a supine position with the legs in the air.

- This many be done from a seated position by bringing the ankle up over the top of the other leg and either leaving that leg on the ground (see Figure 6.82) or lifting the bottom leg to deepen the stretch (see Figure 6.83).

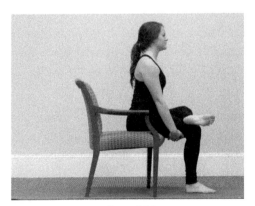

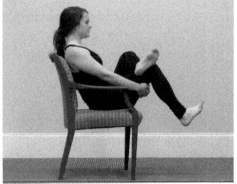

Figure 6.82   *Figure 6.83*

Table Top (Goasana)

Table Top (Goasana) (see Figure 6.84) is a pose that is used as a transition between many floor postures. Table Top (Goasana) helps to realign the spine, as well as to lengthen it. The posture also helps with alignment and providing proprioceptive feedback to hemiparetic limbs.

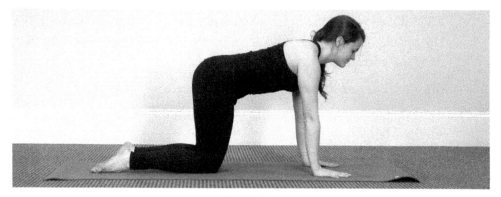

Figure 6.84

Precautions

This pose is contraindicated for carpal tunnel syndrome and injury to the wrists or knees. For clients with stroke who have a dense hemiparalysis, this posture may not be accessible or may only be completed with a lot of assistance from the therapist (or two therapists) and may require the use of a fold-down mat table instead of the floor. Quadruped is commonly included in post-stroke rehabilitation efforts and should be considered when using yoga as well.

Directions

1. Direct the client to come onto all fours. They should place their hands directly under their shoulders, with the palms flat on the ground, and place their knees directly under their hips. The knees should be approximately the width of the hips.

2. They should gaze at the hands, flatten the back, press into the palms, and straighten the back. They should reach the tail energetically towards the back of the room, and the crown of the head towards the front of the room.

Modifications/Props

- A blanket under the knees, folded in thirds, helps to reduce discomfort.

- Instead of having the palms flat on the ground, use fists.

- To make this a balancing posture, raise one arm at a time, while maintaining the integrity of the length of the spine. To further engage the core muscles and challenge, raise the opposite leg simultaneously for a balancing Table Top pose (Goasana). Make sure to repeat on the other side.

- If repetition is not accessible on the other side due to hemiparesis or other impairments, the client may engage in a mental practice by imagining how it would feel to complete the exercise on the opposite side.

- Table Top (Goasana) can be done against the wall instead of on the ground by standing with the feet firmly planted on the ground and arms extended forward with the palms flat against the wall (see Figure 6.85).

- Table Top (Goasana) can be done in a seated position by beginning in seated Mountain pose (Tadasana) and extending the arms directly in front (see Figure 6.86).

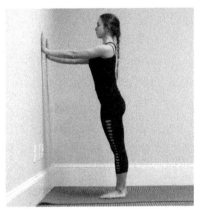

Figure 6.85

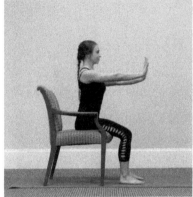

Figure 6.86

Upward Facing Dog (Urdha Mukha Svanasana)

Upward Facing Dog (Urdha Mukha Svanasana) (see Figure 6.87) is a pose that is used in many yoga classes. It has a number of benefits, including improving posture, strengthening the spine, arms, and wrists, and stimulating the abdominal organs. Upward Facing Dog (Urdha Mukha Svanasana) also stretches the upper body and torso. This pose improves alignment of the core body structure and may improve proprioception for a hemiparetic limb.

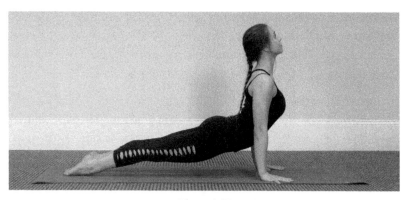

Figure 6.87

Precautions

This pose is contraindicated for people with back injury, carpal tunnel syndrome, or headache.

Directions

1. Direct the client to lie prone on the floor and extend the legs back with the top of the feet resting on the floor.

2. They should bend the elbows and place the palms on the floor under their shoulders. They should inhale, push into the hands, and extend the arms, lifting the trunk and hips off the ground.

3. They should firm the thighs and abdomen, and pull the elbows in towards the waist. They should press the tailbone towards the front of the hips, while lifting the front of the hips towards the belly.

4. They should lift the head towards the ceiling and extend the chest forward, being careful not to push too hard into the lower back.

5. To release, they can roll down gently.

Modifications/Props

*   This pose requires a fair amount of upper-body strength. A bolster or thick, rolled-up blanket under the top of the thighs may help with trunk extension.

*   This can be done by pushing on the seat or back of a chair, holding the back of a chair, or on the wall (see Figure 6.88).

*   The knees can also be down for this pose.

- For extra height, add a bolster under the hips and reach towards the top of the mat.

- This pose could be incorporated into a seated practice and done from a chair (see Figure 6.89).

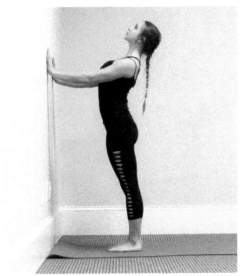

Figure 6.88

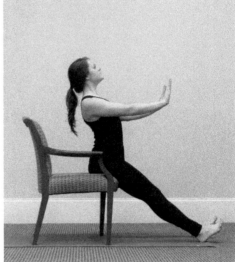

Figure 6.89

Warrior I (Virabhadrasana I)

Warrior I (Virabhadrasana I) (see Figure 6.90) is a strong foundational balancing posture. Warrior I (Virabhadrasana I) helps to relax the mind and body, as well as to strengthen the legs and open the shoulders and chest. This pose also helps to improve concentration and focus. Warrior I (Virabhadrasana I) may stretch the hip flexors, which are often very tight in clients with stroke.

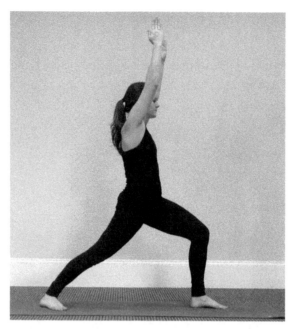

Figure 6.90

Precautions

Individuals with neck problems should keep the head and neck neutral. Individuals with shoulder problems should not raise the arms but instead should use the Prayer pose (Anjali Mudra) for the hands. Raising the arms above the head is contraindicated in individuals with high blood pressure and heart problems.

Directions

1. Direct the client to start in Mountain pose (Tadasana). They should inhale, exhale, and extend the right foot back in a high lunge position, modifying the right foot to extend to the right at a 45–60-degree angle. The left foot should be pointing straight ahead, with the left knee bent and the left foot directly under the left knee.

2. They should rotate the hips and pelvis so they are pointing straight ahead, parallel with the wall in front.

3. They should raise the arms overhead, lifting the ribs away from the pelvis. They should extend energetically through the right foot, lift the torso, and bring the arms overhead. The pinky fingers should turn in towards each other.

4. Ask them to relax the arms and legs, or transition into another pose. Make sure they repeat on the other side.

Modifications/Props

- Step on a sandbag or rolled-up mat to help keep the back foot on the ground.

- The arms may feel more stable in Prayer pose (Anjali Mudra).

- This pose may be done as a seated pose from a chair (see Figure 6.91).

- A chair may help to provide stability. Place it parallel with the front, short side of the mat.

- The asana can be done facing the wall, and placing the hands against the wall for stability (see Figure 6.92).

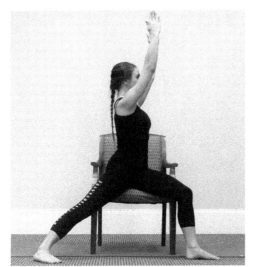

Figure 6.91

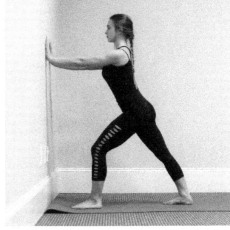

Figure 6.92

Warrior II (Virabhadrasana II)

Warrior II (Virabhadrasana II) (see Figure 6.93) is often done following Warrior I (Virabhadrasana I), but it can be a stand-alone pose. This posture strengthens the upper extremities and opens the chest and shoulders. Warrior II (Virabhadrasana II) also strengthens the lower body and improves concentration and focus. Warrior II (Virabhadrasana II) may stretch the hip flexors and groin muscles, which are often very tight in clients with stroke.

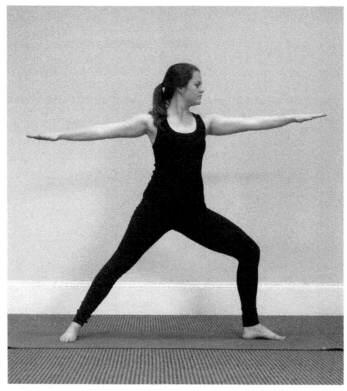

Figure 6.93

Precautions

If neck problems are present, do not look towards the front fingers, but maintain the gaze over the long side of the mat. This pose is contraindicated for individuals with diarrhea and high blood pressure.

Directions

1. Direct the client to start in Mountain pose (Tadasana). They should inhale, exhale, and extend the right foot back in a high lunge position, modifying the right foot to extend to the right at a 90-degree angle. The left foot should be pointing straight ahead, with the left knee bent and the left foot directly under the left knee.

2. They should rotate the hips and pelvis so they are parallel with the long side of the yoga mat.

3. They should extend the arms, so that the left arm is over the left bent knee, and the right arm is over the right straight leg. Ask them to bring the gaze over the middle finger of the left hand, stretch the arms away from each other, and energetically pull the shoulder blades apart from each other.

4. They should relax the arms and legs, or transition into another pose. Make sure they repeat on the other side.

Modifications/Props

- Step on a sandbag or rolled-up mat to help keep the back of the foot on the ground.

- The arms may feel more stable in Prayer pose (Anjali Mudra).

- A chair may help to provide stability. Place it parallel with the long side of the mat.

- This pose could be conducted from a seated position (see Figure 6.94).

- This pose can be done with the back up against the wall for stability and to help feel the alignment (see Figure 6.95).

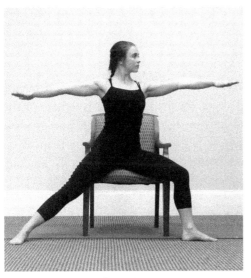

Figure 6.94

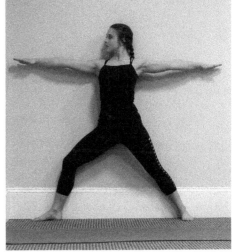

Figure 6.95

Warrior III (Virabhadrasana III)

Warrior III (Virabhadrasana III) (see Figure 6.96) is a challenging balancing pose, and it can be done in transition from Warrior I or II (Virabhadrasana I or II) or as a stand-alone pose. Warrior III (Virabhadrasana III) strengthens the lower body and expands and strengthens the shoulders and upper body. This pose also tightens the core and improves balance and posture.

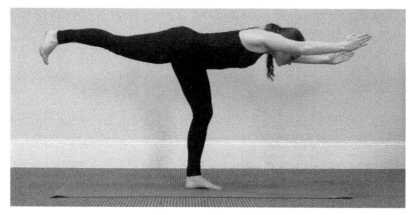

Figure 6.96

Precautions

Warrior III (Virabhadrasana III) is contraindicated for individuals with high blood pressure and will likely be very difficult for clients with lower extremity hemiparesis.

Directions

1. Direct the client to start in Mountain pose (Tadasana). They should inhale, bend the knees slightly, and exhale. Ask them to shift the weight into the left leg, begin to lean forward, and let the right leg raise in a straight line behind the body. They should ensure that the left foot is firmly planted on the ground and the toes of the right foot are pointing down towards the floor. The torso should be parallel to the floor.

2. They should bring the arms forward so they extend next to the ears and are parallel to each other. Ask them to energetically imagine that the arms are being pulled to the front of the room while the lifted foot is being pulled towards the back of the room. Ask them to energetically imagine energy coursing from the torso into the standing leg, while squeezing the thighs together.

3. They should ensure that the hips are parallel to the floor. The gaze should be forward.

4. Ask them to release, and repeat on the other side.

Modifications/Props

• This posture can be done by holding on to the top of the chair instead of the arms extending forward (see Figure 6.97).

• This posture can be done with the hands on the wall for stability (see Figure 6.98).

- Position a chair in front of the standing leg, with the seat away from the individual, for additional stability.

- This posture could be completed with the standing leg slightly bent, to increase stability.

- The arms can be in Prayer pose (Anjali Mudra).

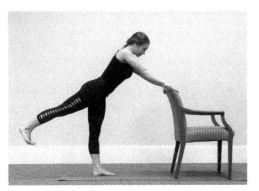 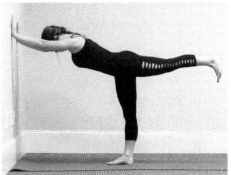

Figure 6.97   *Figure 6.98*

Wide Legged Forward Fold (Prasarita Padottanasana)

Wide Legged Forward Fold (Prasarita Padottanasana) (see Figure 6.99) is an inverted balancing pose.

Forward folds are known to calm the brain and stretch the back of the legs (including the hamstrings and calves), while strengthening the front of the leg (including the thighs and knees). Forward folds may also reduce fatigue and anxiety and reduce headaches.

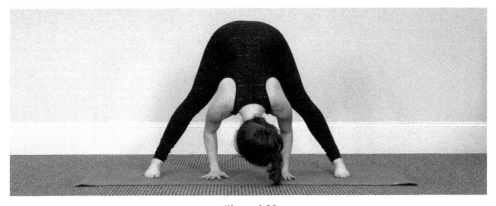

Figure 6.99

Precautions

For individuals with high blood pressure or lower back problems, avoid the full forward fold and use the modification shown in Figure 6.101.

Directions

1. Direct the client to stand in Mountain pose (Tadasana) facing the long side of the mat.

2. They should extend the feet towards the edges of the mat, approximately four feet apart.

3. They should bring the hands to the hips, raise the arches of the feet, draw them upward, and root down through the four corners of the feet.

4. They should bend the knees slightly and lower the torso towards the floor.

5. They should extend the arms towards the floor. The arms and legs should be perpendicular to the floor. Ask them to push the top of the quadriceps back to elongate the torso (taking care to not lock the knees) and draw the thighs away from each other.

6. To release, they can bend the knees slightly, place the hands on the hips, and raise the head and torso.

Modifications/Props

- The arms can rest on two blocks—each placed under the head in a comfortable position approximately shoulder distance apart (see Figure 6.100).

- Props can be built up so that the head rests on the props.

- This pose can easily be done standing at the wall to avoid a full forward fold (see Figure 6.101).

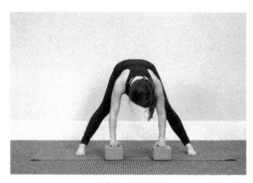

Figure 6.100

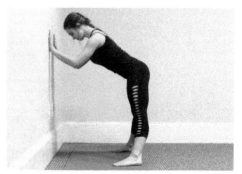

Figure 6.101

Additionally, there are movements that are not traditional yoga poses but are included in the practice sequences.

CHAPTER 7

Descriptions and Modifications of Restorative Asana (Postures) for Yoga Post-Stroke

Introduction

As we have mentioned in this book several times, while there is a very important need for the use of physically active, stimulating asanas and yoga practice (as identified in the previous chapter), there is an equivalent need for relaxation so that the body and mind have time to heal. Allowing the mind and body to heal may further enhance post-stroke recovery. Restorative yoga has been said to support the immune system, soothe the nervous system, relieve stress, regulate blood pressure, enhance mental and physical health, improve concentration and clarity, and enhance recovery from illness. However, in our fast-paced culture, it is often difficult for individuals to feel that relaxation is a worthy endeavor. When we do not relax and restore, we are unable to best complete the tasks we have or our daily responsibilities. Burdens, stressors, and associated toxins build up. Add to that mix a cerebral infarct, or stroke, and the need for the body to relax and restore itself is multiplied! Also consider the acute or rehabilitation environments. These environments are inherently stressful! Rehabilitation environments are commonly loud, bright, noisy environments where, suddenly, others are directing an individual's care. For many, this may be terrifying, stressful, and overwhelming. Offering a place and space for respite, such as restorative yoga, is a balm for clients and their family members.

Teaching restorative classes is different than teaching more traditional physically active yoga classes in a number of ways. During restorative yoga classes or sessions, postures are held for up to 20 minutes, and the individual in the pose is fully supported by the props.

In this chapter, we will review the restorative asanas that are identified in the sample restorative sequences found in Chapter 12. Like the format in Chapter 6, for each pose we include the common or English translation of the name, the Sanskrit name (if available, although it seems that many restorative poses do not have a Sanskrit name), any known precautions for the pose, directions to instruct the asana, and how to transition out of the pose. Modifications and props are not specifically identified here, as in all restorative poses the pose should be modified (with props) until the individual is comfortable and can maintain the pose. There should be no pain or discomfort in restorative yoga poses—these poses are solely for relaxation. Experiment with the use of all props—there are so many ways to modify postures to enhance comfort. Do not be afraid of trying new things and new ways to modify the poses or use the props.

Props

As mentioned, props can and should be used to support the client. Each prop can be used in a variety of ways to support the client, and it is important to practice or explore the placement of the props to determine what feels best for the client. Typical props used in restorative poses include bolsters, blocks, sandbags, eye pillows, straps, and blankets. Here we describe some of the ways the props can be used, but, again, it is important to play around with them to see what works best!

Bolsters

Bolsters come in a variety of sizes—large and round, small and round, or a flatter, more rectangular version. Bolsters can be placed under the knees in any supine pose to reduce strain on the back, or in many poses to provide support or comfort. See Figure 7.1 for a picture of flat and round bolsters.

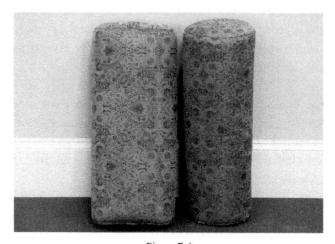

Figure 7.1

Blocks

Blocks are typically made of rubber, cork, or wood. Clearly, each material differs in pliability and strength. Blocks also come in a wide width (approximately 4 inches) or a narrower width (approximately 3 inches). Blocks can be used at three heights: short, medium, or tall. Some types of blocks feel better under parts of the body than others. For example, when using a block under the hips, some prefer a rubber block that has a little more give than a wood block, which has no give. See Figure 7.2 for a picture of blocks at different heights.

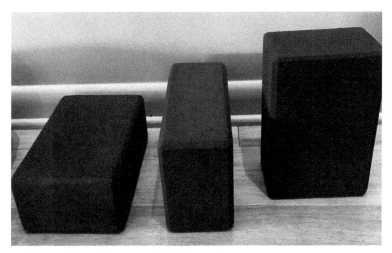

Figure 7.2

Sandbags

Sandbags can be used to provide grounding or weight to a body part. Some people really enjoy the feel of a sandbag on their pelvis during supine postures, while other people can't stand this feeling! Make sure to ask your client's permission prior to placing a sandbag, particularly in the pelvic region. Sandbags, when placed on a spastic limb, can weight the arm and encourage it to relax. Sandbags can also be placed on feet to encourage the feet to feel more grounded. See Figure 7.3 for a picture of a sandbag.

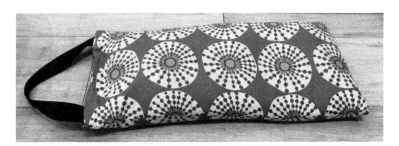

Figure 7.3

Eye Pillows

Eye pillows are used in supine positions to help promote relaxation and comfort. Make sure to ask your client for permission before placing an eye pillow on them and consider asking them to remove their glasses (or ask if you can do this) so they feel the gentle weight of the eye pillow on their eyes. Some eye pillows are gently scented with essential oils, so make sure your client does not have an allergy or sensitivity to the scent prior to use. See Figure 7.4 for a picture of an eye pillow.

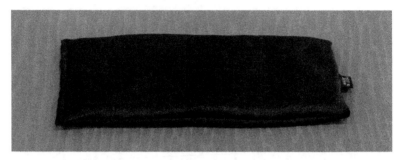

Figure 7.4

Yoga Straps

Yoga straps are used to bind parts of the body or to help extend the length of the arms so that postures that require a lot of flexibility are more accessible. Yoga straps differ in length, and typically have a buckle. These buckles are usually mode of metal or plastic. A gait belt can be used instead of a yoga strap, but a yoga strap can never be used instead of a gait belt! See Figure 7.5 for a picture of a yoga strap.

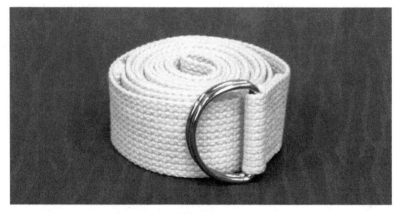

Figure 7.5

Blankets

Blankets are widely used in yoga, particularly in restorative postures. Blankets can be rolled in a variety of ways, as demonstrated in Figures 7.6–7.9. A flat, unrolled blanket that is folded can also be used to provide gentle support. Blankets are a nice option to use when a soft support is needed. And, of course, a blanket can be used to cover your client in a supine posture, as temperature regulation may be an issue following a stroke. Blankets are really versatile in their use; try adding them to poses to see if they make a difference for your client.

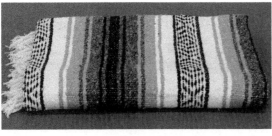

Figure 7.6

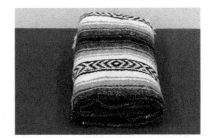

Figure 7.8

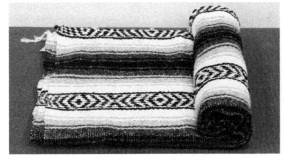

Figure 7.7

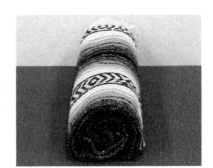

Figure 7.9

A Few Notes About Restorative Postures

- All postures will be done on a solid surface. They can be done on the floor, on a mat table, or on the bed.

- Unless otherwise noted, postures should be held for five to ten minutes.

- If a twist is involved, make sure that the client engages in the posture on both sides to ensure that the sides are evenly stretched.

- The yoga or rehabilitation therapist should instruct the client about where the props should be placed. If the client needs assistance, ask their permission to place the props on or around their body. Never remove or place anything on the client's body without their permission.

Basic Relaxation Asana

This is a supine pose that resembles Corpse pose (Savasana). It can be an unexpected and rewarding way to start a yoga practice (as used in Restorative Practice 1, Chapter 12). This pose lowers the blood pressure and heart rate, releases muscular tension, reduces fatigue, improves sleep, enhances immune response, and helps to manage chronic pain. This asana quiets the frontal lobes of the brain. See Figures 7.10–7.12 for three variations of the Basic Relaxation Asana. This pose can be held for up to 20 minutes.

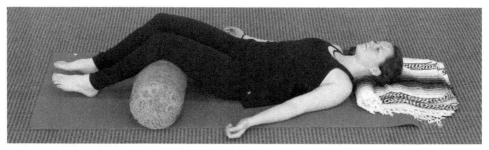

Figure 7.10

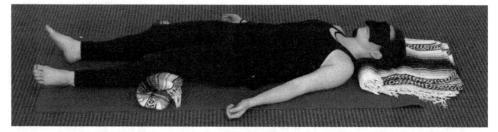

Figure 7.11

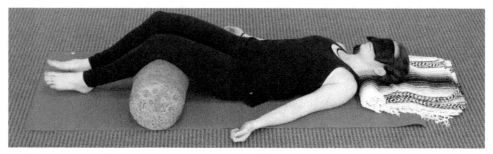

Figure 7.12

Precautions
No specific precautions noted.

Directions

1. Have your client start supine in Corpse pose (Savasana) with their arms out in a T and knees bent and supported on a rolled-up blanket or bolster.

2. Have a second blanket under the head/neck, rolled in thirds, with the largest part of the roll under the neck.

3. Adjust the prop placement so that the neck is comfortable.

4. The chin should be slightly lower than the forehead.

5. It may feel good for the client to rest each arm on a blanket that is also folded.

6. If the client gets cold, a blanket covering the body may be helpful.

7. An eye pillow may facilitate relaxation.

8. A sandbag could be placed parallel with the waistband of the pants over the pelvic region.

Transition

To transition from the Basic Relaxation Asana, the therapist or client should remove the props, and the client should bend their knees, roll to the right side of their body, and pause. The client should push themselves up to a seated position (with assistance if needed).

Cat Cow (Chakravakasana) (Upright Seated Cat (Marjariasana) and Cow (Bitilasana))

This pose is composed of two poses that are frequently joined together because they flow well together with the breath. Cat pose (Marjariasana) (see Figure 7.13) and Cow pose (Bitilasana) (see Figure 7.14) combined make Cat Cow (Chakravakasana). Cat Cow (Chakravakasana) is a gentle stretch for the back, trunk, and neck, and is thought to reduce back pain. It creates space for the vertebrae. These asanas can be completed in an upright, seated position, for a restorative version of the pose.

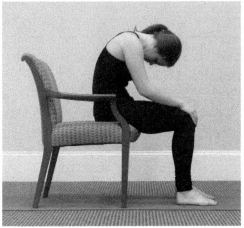
Figure 7.13

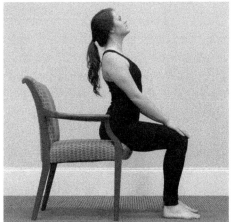
Figure 7.14

Precautions

For individuals with lower back problems, only perform Cow pose (Bitilasana) and then return the body to neutral instead of flowing to Cat pose (Marjariasana).

Directions

1. Have your client start seated in Easy pose (Sukhasana). Their eyes can be open or closed.

2. Ask your client to inhale and tilt their pelvis forward. The client should raise their chest and point the chin at a 70-degree angle. They should hold for three seconds.

3. During this posture, the client should rest their hands on their knees.

4. Ask your client to exhale and curve their spine. Their chin should point towards the navel.

5. Encourage the client to synchronize the breath so that the exhalation occurs with the Cat (Marjariasana) part (chest forward, chin up) and inhalation occurs with the Cow (Bitilasana) part (chin tucked, back rounded).

6. Continue for five rotations of Upright Seated Cat (Marjariasana) and Cow (Bitilasana).

Transition

Ask your client to inhale deeply and exhale fully. Ask them to open their eyes if they are closed.

Corpse Pose (Savasana)

The Corpse pose (Savasana) is one of the most important postures because it allows the mind and body to rest after a physical asana practice. The pose allows the individual to soak in the benefits of the asanas that have preceded it. Corpse pose (Savasana) is thought to reduce blood pressure, calm the mind, and enhance relaxation throughout the body. It also reduces headache, fatigue, and insomnia. See Figures 7.15–7.18 for several variations of Corpse pose (Savasana). This pose can be held for up to 20 minutes.

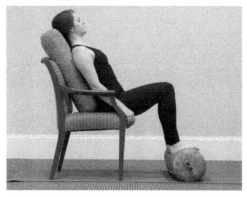

Figure 7.15

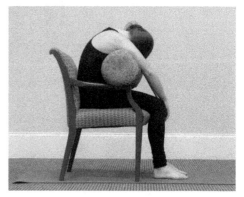

Figure 7.16

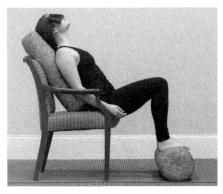

Figure 7.17

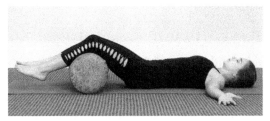

Figure 7.18

Precautions

Laying in supine position can strain the lower back, so placing a bolster or rolled-up blanket underneath the knees helps to reduce that strain.

Directions

1. Instruct your client to extend their body in a supine position. Instead of laying supine on the floor, some may prefer to recline with a bolster under their knees.

2. Depending on your client's preference, a rolled-up blanket can be placed under the neck and/or head.

3. The client's arms can be placed at their side or overhead, depending on individual preference. The palms should be placed face up. Ensure that the shoulder blades are both resting on the floor.

4. The client's legs should be extended straight out in front of their body, with the legs abducted towards the width of the mat, with the feet turned out if that feels comfortable. A bolster under the knees may reduce strain on the lower back. The knees can also stay bent, and a strap can bind the thighs.

5. Encourage your client to extend their neck and head towards the top of the mat.

6. Sandbags can be placed on the different limbs or pelvic area to provide a feeling of grounding.

7. Encourage your client to soften their face and close their eyes if that feels comfortable. Ask them to relax the tongue, relax the cheeks, and soften the eyes.

8. A guideline for the length of time to spend in this pose is to practice it for five minutes for every 30 minutes of physical practice.

Transition

To release, ask the client to bring the attention back to the room. Have them roll on to their right side and press their body up with the head coming up last.

Queen's Pose (Salamba Baddha Konasana)

This is a reclining pose that feels as if the individual is resting on a throne. This pose opens the back and the pelvic region. This pose should be held for around ten minutes. See Figures 7.19–7.21 for pictures of the Queen's pose (Salamba Baddha Konasana) with several variations.

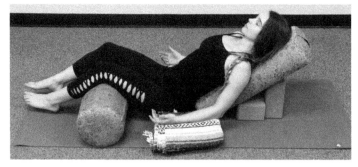

Figure 7.19

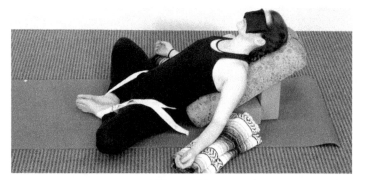

Figure 7.20

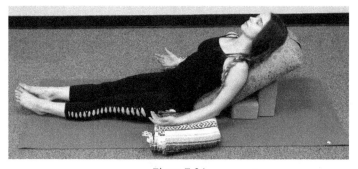

Figure 7.21

Precautions

The client should use caution when descending on to the bolster. It may be easier for them to start on their side and scoot on top of the bolster, instead of lowering down to it. Also, if the strap is placed to provide support for the knees, ensure that it is not so tight that it will cause discomfort but not so loose that it does not provide any support.

Directions

1. Place a small block at the head of the mat with a tall block behind it (or adjust the blocks to short, medium, or tall heights as needed or desired based on comfort).

2. Place a bolster lengthwise over the blocks.

3. Have the client start with their head towards the top of the mat and position their hips at the base of the bolster. Have the client bend their knees with their feet planted on the ground, or their legs can be extended straight ahead.

4. Ask your client to recline backwards over the bolster (and assist as needed). Adjust the incline to high or low as needed by changing the height of the blocks.

5. Rolled-up blankets or small bolsters can be placed under each arm to provide support.

6. For added comfort, add a blanket doubled under the hips.

7. Add an eye pillow if desired.

8. Add a sandbag to the pelvic region if desired, or put it on top of the feet if the feet are planted on the ground with the knees bent.

9. Encourage the client to rest quietly.

Transition

Ask your client to roll to their right side and come to an upright seated position.

Reclining Twist with a Bolster

This asana is thought to reduce strain in the back and the intercostal muscles. As the muscles relax, breathing is enhanced. See Figures 7.22 and 7.23 for examples of Reclining Twist with a Bolster. This pose should be held for five to ten minutes on each side.

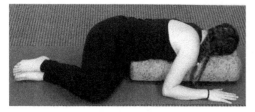

Figure 7.22

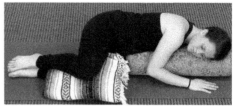

Figure 7.23

Precautions

Individuals with disc disease, sacroiliac problems, or other spinal conditions should proceed with great care. If twisting is uncomfortable or contraindicated, the client can recline on the bolster without adding the twist.

Directions

1. Have the client position their body so that the right hip is resting on the floor. Their knees should be stacked on top of each other (relatively).

2. Place the bolster so it is touching the client's left hip, pointing away from the body toward the top of the mat (the bolster is placed behind the individual). Twist the torso toward the bolster and have them recline on it until the entire weight of the body is supported. The twist can be eliminated if this feels more comfortable to the client.

3. A blanket rolled in thirds can be placed at the top of the bolster for support of the head.

4. The client's arms can drape to the side of the bolster.

5. If the client's top knee is uncomfortable or lifted, a folded blanket could be fitted to fill this space.

Transition

To transition from this pose, encourage your client to push up and come into a seated position.

Restorative Child's Pose on Bolsters (Restorative Balasana)

Child's pose (Balasana) engages the parasympathetic nervous system and encourages the relaxation response. This pose also reduces strain in the neck, back, and hips, and calms the mind. Child's pose (Balasana) helps relieve anxiety, stress, and fatigue. This pose can be held for five minutes on each side. See Figures 7.24–7.26 for pictures of several versions of this pose.

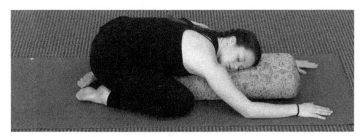

Figure 7.24

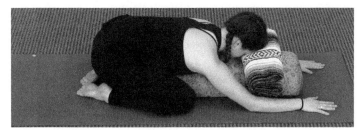

Figure 7.25

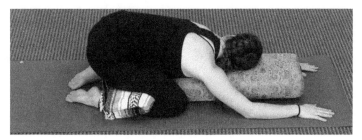

Figure 7.26

Precautions

If a knee injury is present, avoid or modify this pose. To modify this pose, a bolster can be placed over the heels so that the amount of knee flexion is greatly reduced. This pose is contraindicated for people with diarrhea.

Directions

1. Place one or two bolsters on top of each other (or mix in some blankets to get the height just right—there should be no straining, just pure relaxation) in the center of the mat.

2. Ask your client to come into Child's pose (Balasana) with their knees straddling the end of the bolsters. To do this follow these steps:

i. The client comes into Table Top (Goasana). Have them bring their toes together (or as close as is comfortable) and bring their hips towards the heels. Ask them to separate the knees as wide as is comfortable—about the width of the hips.

ii. Have the client relax their torso on top of their thighs. Encourage them to think about pushing the hips towards the heels. You can give your client a nice visual by saying, "Imagine a long, stretched-out line between the top of the head and the bottom of the sacrum."

3. If this is uncomfortable for the knees, a blanket or bolster placed between the calves and hamstrings can reduce the pressure.

4. Encourage your client to relax their torso onto the bolsters, resting their head on one cheek. If this is uncomfortable, the client can rest their head on a rolled-up blanket, placed midway on the bolster.

5. Your client's arms can rest at their sides or in front of their body—whichever is more comfortable.

6. At five minutes, ask them to turn their head to switch cheeks.

Transition

To release, encourage your client to raise their torso to come into a seated position.

Seated Bound Angle Pose (Baddha Konasana)

This upright posture uses blocks to support the knees and increase the comfort in the seated position. Because of the properties of this asana, there is a good opportunity to engage the Dhyana Mudra to enhance the therapeutic benefits. See Figure 7.27 for a picture of Seated Bound Angle pose (Baddha Konasana). Hold this pose for up to ten minutes.

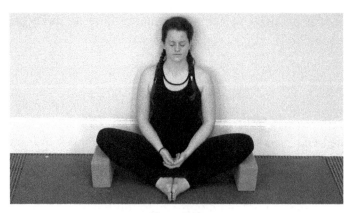

Figure 7.27

Precautions

None noted.

Directions

1. Place a blanket or bolster (depending on the flexibility in the hips and the client's comfort level) for the client to sit on.

2. Ask your client to come to a seated pose on the blanket or bolster with their back against a wall.

3. Have the client bend the knees in front of the body, bringing the feet together and letting the knees open with the soles of the feet touching. The heels can be up to 12 inches away from the groin area, depending on the comfort in the knees.

4. Place a bolster or block under each knee.

5. Place the hands in Dhyana Mudra (pictured in Chapter 10). The Dhyana Mudra involves both hands working together, with the tips of each thumb touching while the left fingers are cradling the right hand (which is facing up), and with both hands sitting in the lap.

6. Ask the client to close their eyes and breathe gently and slowly.

Transition

Release the blocks.

Side Resting Pose with Bolster

This asana provides stimulation for the abdominal organs and relaxation for the nervous systems. It also provides relief for fatigue and high blood pressure. This pose can be held for up to ten minutes on each side. See Figure 7.28 for a picture of this pose.

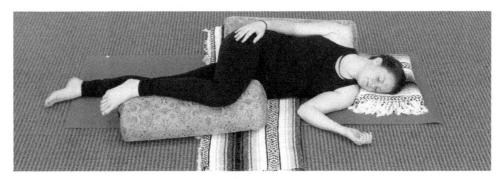

Figure 7.28

Precautions

None noted.

Directions

1. Place a blanket that has been folded over twice parallel with the edge of the short end of the mat towards the top of the mat. Fold another blanket in half and place it on the mat.

2. Have the client lay down on their right side and position the bolster between the legs, with the left leg draped over the bolster, as comfortable. A blanket under the foot that is on the ground may increase comfort.

3. Place a bolster in front of the abdomen and another resting against the back of the torso.

4. Encourage your client to choose a comfortable position for their arms—potentially using the right arm as a pillow or placing the arm under the body.

5. After five minutes, encourage the client to push their body up to a seated position, and lie down on the other side.

Transition

Encourage the client to use their bottom arm to push their body up to a seated position.

Supported Reclining Bound Angle Pose (Supta Baddha Konasana)

Supported Reclining Bound Angle pose (Supta Baddha Konasana) is one of the most important poses in the restorative series. It opens the chest, abdomen, and pelvis. These areas are often restricted by the ways we stand and sit, the shape of our chairs, and the fit of our clothes. This pose also lowers blood pressure and helps with breathing problems. Following a stroke, individuals tend to spend a lot of time in a seated position. This pose can help to address some of the discomfort caused by so much time spent sitting down. It is also helpful for women during their menstrual cycle and during menopause. As the chest opens, the arms and legs are cradled by the props. See Figure 7.29 for a picture of this pose.

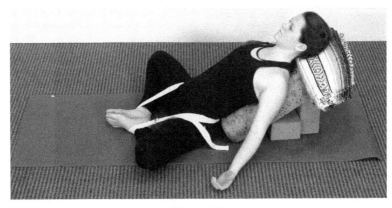

Figure 7.29

Precautions

Encourage the client to use caution when descending to the bolster (and assist as needed). It may be easier for them to start on their side and scoot on top of the bolster, instead of lowering down to it.

Directions

1. This reclining pose starts with a similar set up to Queen's pose (Salamba Baddha Konasana). Place a small block at the head of the mat with a tall block behind it (or adjusting the blocks to short, medium, or tall heights as needed or desired, based on comfort).

2. Place a bolster lengthwise over the blocks.

3. Roll a blanket and place it at the top of the bolster to support the head.

4. Ask your client to place their hips at the base of the bolster. If there is any discomfort in the lower back, adjust the height of the support by adding blankets or decrease the height by using a blanket instead of a bolster.

5. Ask your client to recline backwards over the bolster (and assist as needed). Adjust the incline to high or low as needed by changing the height of the blocks.

6. After the client has reclined, ask them to plant their feet on the floor and open the knees. Blocks can be placed under the knees or a strap can be placed around the back, under the knees, and over the feet (see Figure 7.29).

7. Place a rolled-up blanket under each arm for support.

8. The forehead should be higher than the chin, the chin should be higher than the breastbone, and the breastbone should be higher than the pubic bone.

9. For added comfort, add a doubled blanket under the hips.

10. Add an eye pillow if desired.

11. Add a sandbag to the pelvic region if desired, or put it on top of the feet if the feet are planted on the ground with the knees bent.

12. Encourage the client to rest quietly.

Transition

Ask your client to pull on the strap to bring the knees together. You can assist the client by releasing the strap. Encourage the client to come to a seated position and extend the legs. It may feel good for them to shake their legs out.

Supported Wide-Angle Seated Forward Bend (Upavistha Konasana)

The point of this pose is not to stretch but to open the hamstrings and lower back, so all modifications should be made with comfort in mind. Forward bending postures quiet the organs of digestion and elimination, such as the stomach, intestines, and liver. This pose can be held for up to ten minutes and can be seen in Figures 7.30 and 7.31.

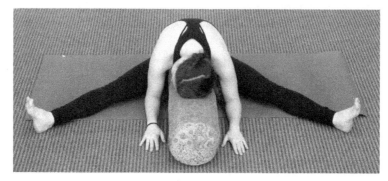

Figure 7.30

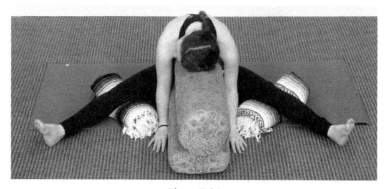

Figure 7.31

Precautions

Some individuals do not find forward folds restorative, instead they find them to be quite unpleasant. If their primary discomfort comes from tight hamstrings, this can be modified, as noted below. Check in with your client about their comfort in the pose.

Directions

1. Encourage your client to sit on the floor or mat table with their legs apart and one or two bolsters between the legs. If their knees feel uncomfortable, encourage your client to bring their legs closer until the discomfort subsides and they feel the stretch only in their inner thighs. It is also possible to add a small blanket under each knee if the discomfort is felt in the knees.

2. A blanket under their sit bones may enhance feelings of comfort.

3. Once they are comfortably seated, encourage your client to lean forward and rest their torso, arms, and head on the bolster. Their head can rest on their forearms, with the arms resting on the bolster.

Transition

Bend the knees. Slowly raise the torso.

CHAPTER 8

Descriptions of Pranayama (Breath Work) Used in Yoga Post-Stroke

Introduction

In Sanskrit, "prana" means breath or life force and "ayama" means restrain or control; thus the term "pranayama" can be translated to "breath control." Pranayama, or breath work, is an important part of yoga practice, and it can be used as a stand-alone practice as well. Pranayama is one of the eight limbs of yoga. After a stroke, an individual may not feel that they have much control over their body—maybe they've lost some or all function on one side, or maybe their thoughts are fuzzy and unclear. A practice focused on breath work can provide a sense of control for the individual, as this is one ability that everyone has. Breath is something that we take for granted, but learning to breathe with intention is the fourth limb of yoga and can be an important tool in recovery of mind and body health.

In our research, we had several individuals whose vision improved substantially following the eight-week yoga intervention. They reported to us that their neuro-ophthalmologists thought that the focus on breath work was essential in their vision changes. When we spoke at greater length with our yoga therapist about the potential mechanisms for the vision changes, she identified having chosen pranayama that are hypothesized to activate the bilateral hemispheres of the brain, such as Alternate Nostril Breathing (Nadi Shodhana Pranayama, described below). While we do not know specifically that pranayama was responsible for increased vision, other researchers have reported that a regular pranayama practice: improves mood by reducing depression and anxiety; reduces blood pressure and stress; and increases energy and relaxation in the muscles (Sengupta, 2012).

In Chapter 5, we provided a brief review of the autonomic nervous system. There we saw that the autonomic nervous system was made of the sympathetic and parasympathetic nervous systems. The sympathetic nervous system triggers the fight-or-flight response, and when this occurs the breath becomes shallow and rapid, which, along with the other physiological changes during this experience, allows the individual to react quickly to the stressor. A pranayama practice that focuses on the opposite of shallow and rapid breathing—namely deep breathing—can assist in activating the parasympathetic nervous system, or the relaxation response. When deep, slow, and steady breathing is performed, the vagus nerve is stimulated, which reduces blood pressure, slows the heart rate, and calms the body and mind.

The pranayama practices and techniques described in this chapter can be used to activate the sympathetic or parasympathetic nervous systems and are divided below as "Pranayama for Relaxation" and "Pranayama for Alertness."

Tips for Teaching the Practice of Pranayama

- Unless otherwise noted, pranayama is typically practiced in Easy pose (Sukhasana), with the spine erect and in a comfortable seated position. In Easy pose (Sukhasana), the weight should be equally applied to the sit bones (the ischial tuberosities). For individuals with stroke, it is appropriate to modify the seat as needed by using yoga or therapy props to ensure an appropriate seated position. Many pranayama can also be practiced in a chair, with the feet resting on the floor. If necessary, pranayama can also be taught in bed, although an upright position is best (unless otherwise indicated).

- Good posture is important for reaping the benefits of pranayama. Instruct your client that in addition to the weight being on the sit bones, attention should be paid to the area that exists between the sit bones and the bottom of the rib cage, and cue them to elongate this space. A focus on straightening or centering the ribs over the pelvis will promote a good sitting posture. It may be beneficial for your client to sit on a blanket or bolster if it enhances comfort and ease in sitting. Next, direct your client's attention between the bottom of the ribs and the top of the ribs. The top of the ribs to the crown of the head is the final section of the body for your client to concentrate on elongating when working on enhancing the sitting posture. This seated position allows the energy to flow freely throughout the body.

- Ensure that your client practices pranayama on an empty-ish stomach. A full belly makes focusing on breath work difficult, as respiration is influenced by digestion.

- Encourage your client to try to remain relaxed during pranayama practice. Ask your client to notice the muscles of the face, eyes, cheeks, skin, tongue, throat, and lips, and not to stiffen or tense these unless instructed to do so.

- Remind your client to stay cognizant about the sound of the breath. Praise audible breath: audible breathing is beautiful and a good way to regulate the practice.

- Finally, encourage your client to only do pranayama that feel good. Ask for feedback about each pranayama that you teach, and do not force or instruct pranayama that promote anxiety or discomfort for your client. There are many choices for good breathing practices, so help your client choose a practice that feels good.

- In the descriptions of each pranayama below, the ideal length of time or number of repetitions from a yogic perspective is provided. However, the yoga or rehabilitation therapist should consider reducing the amount of time or repetitions used with a client, based on the client's ability level, dexterity, and mood. It is also important, unless otherwise noted, to do the same number of repetitions on both the left and right sides.

Pranayama for Relaxation
Alternate Nostril Breathing (Nadi Shodhana Pranayama)

Alternate Nostril Breathing (Nadi Shodhana Pranayama, pronounced "notti shaadna") is a powerful breathing practice that is important to connect the bilateral hemispheres of the brain, which can develop the left and right sides of the brain and may balance the impaired side of the body. This is a powerful pranayama that can be used in acute care or chronic phases of stroke recovery. Nadi is a Sanskrit term that means "channel" or "flow," and Shodhana means "purification"; thus this pranayama is thought to purify the channels of the body while connecting and balancing the left and right hemispheres of the brain.

Precautions

This pranayama involves slight breath retention. Avoid if there is severe or uncontrolled asthma or heart conditions.

Directions

1. Instruct your client to sit comfortably on the floor (the seat or back can be supported with props), a chair with the feet resting on the floor (or blocks if the legs are not long enough to reach the floor), or other comfortable surface, including a bed if the client is not able to transfer out of the bed.

2. Ask the client to allow the spine to lengthen so that the back is straight, the neck is long, and the head is centered over the torso. Encourage the client to close their eyes.

3. Encourage a few rounds of gentle yet deep inhalations and exhalations.

4. Instruct the client to fold the index and middle fingers to touch the base of the right thumb. With the hand in this position, place the right thumb touching the side of the right nostril, and the ring finger on the outside of the left nostril. Stroke-related hemiparesis may lead to decreased dexterity. If the mudra is too complicated or requires too much dexterity, the right nostril can be closed by the thumb of the right hand, and the left nostril closed by the pinky and ring fingers of the same hand.

5. Instruct the client to use the right thumb to close the right nostril (see Figure 8.1). State "Exhale gently, but fully, through the left nostril. Keeping the right nostril closed with the thumb of the right hand, inhale through the left nostril deeply." As the client inhales, ask them to "Encourage the breath to travel upward along the left side of the body—from the root chakra or pelvic floor, up through the organs of reproduction and elimination, through the left kidney, the spleen, the left lung, the heart, and up through the left side of the throat, face, and head. Pause at the crown chakra, or the top of the head."

6. Instruct the client to use the pinky and ring fingers of the right hand to gently close the left nostril and to simultaneously release the right nostril, exhaling fully through the right nostril (see Figure 6.2). State to your client "Let the breath travel down the right side of the body—starting at the crown chakra, to the right side of the head, face, and throat, down the right side of the spine through the heart, the right lung, the liver, the right kidney, the organs of reproduction and elimination, and down to the pelvic floor and root chakra. Pause gently at the bottom of the exhalation."

7. Repeat the same steps, starting with the left nostril. Instruct the client to "Keep the left nostril closed with the pinky and ring finger, inhale deeply through the right nostril, drawing the breath upward along the right side of the body—from the root chakra or pelvic floor, up through the organs of reproduction and elimination, through the right kidney, the spleen, the right lung, the heart, and up through the right side of the throat, face, and head. Pause at the crown chakra or the top of your head."

8. Encourage the client to "Close the right nostril with the thumb, and release air through the left nostril. Exhale fully through the left nostril. Let the breath travel down the left side of the body—starting at the crown chakra, to the left side of the head, face, and throat, down the left side of the spine through the heart, the left lung, the liver, the left kidney, the organs of reproduction and elimination, and down to the pelvic floor and root chakra. Pause gently at the bottom of the exhalation."

9. This completes one round of Alternate Nostril Breathing (Nadi Shodhana Pranayama). Start with one or two cycles to see how your client tolerates this and build from there to up to 10–15 minutes. Note: After the client becomes proficient and comfortable with inhaling and exhaling through the nostrils, a rhythm or count of four for the inhalation, exhalation, and pausing between the inhalations and exhalations can be implemented. This ratio can also be increased as tolerated.

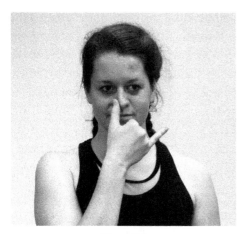

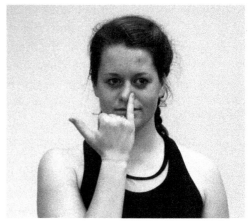

Figure 8.1   *Figure 8.2*

At the end of the Alternate Nostril Breathing practice, suggest that the client releases the right arm and takes several full, deep breaths. This practice can be used at the beginning or end of class or therapy session to promote centering, relaxation, and grounding.

Bee Breath (Bhramari Pranayama)

Bee Breath (Bhramari Pranayama) is a fun and rewarding pranayama practice. This pranayama helps to decrease agitation, frustration, and anxiety, as well as anger. This pranayama has an audible exhale that may produce a tingling sensation on the lips. The sound produced by this pranayama is much like the sound of a bee (fun fact: Bhramari is a type of bee in India).

Precautions

No precautions or contraindications are noted for this pranayama.

Directions

1. Instruct your client to sit comfortably on the floor (the seat or back can be supported with props), a chair with the feet resting on the floor (or blocks if the legs are not long enough to reach the floor), or other comfortable surface, including a bed if the client is not able to transfer out of the bed.

2. Ask the client to allow the spine to lengthen, so that the back is straight, the neck is long, and the head is centered over the torso. Encourage the client to close their eyes and notice their breath.

3. Request that they inhale deeply. Instruct the client to keep the mouth closed on the exhale and make the sound of a bee buzzing around. This may tickle the lips or make someone feel self-conscious, but these sensations pass quickly.

4. The therapist may need to encourage the client to "buzz" more loudly, as people often feel a little self-conscious about making an audible sound.

In some yogic traditions, they place the index fingers between the cheek and ear in Step 3 to make the sounds and vibrations feel deeper and more internalized. This pranayama can be practiced with or without the fingers in the ear. It can also be practiced on the back in supine position or in a chair.

Equal Breaths (Sama Vritti)

Equal Breaths (Sama Vritti) is a pranayama that is simple and easy to practice. As the name implies, this practice requires inhalations and exhalations that are of equal length.

Precautions

Equal Breaths (Sama Vritti) involves some breath retention (kumbhaka), although this is gentle and could be minimized through smaller ratios of retention (for example, for two seconds). Breath retention is contraindicated for individuals who have high blood pressure, heart disease, or abdominal pain.

Directions

1. Instruct your client to sit comfortably on the floor (the seat or back can be supported with props), a chair with the feet resting on the floor (or blocks if the legs are not long enough to reach the floor), or other comfortable surface, including a bed if the client is not able to transfer out of the bed.

2. Ask the client to allow the spine to lengthen, so that the back is straight, the neck is long, and the head is centered over the torso. Encourage the client to close their eyes and notice the breath. Ask them not to change anything but just to notice how it feels in the body. Stay here for approximately five breaths.

3. On your client's inhalation, encourage them to count slowly to three for the length of the inhale and to hold the breath at the top of the inhalation for a moment.

4. Encourage an exhalation for a count of three, with a pause at the bottom of the exhalation.

5. Encourage your client to continue with this pattern for several minutes. It is possible to change the number of seconds counted depending on the individual. Typically, Equal Breaths (Sama Vritti) is counted in threes, fours, fives, or sevens for beginners.

Equal Breaths (Sama Vritti) can be used at the beginning or end of class, to help center the individual, or during class, to help calm or reduce stress if necessary.

Three-Part Breath (Dirga Pranayama)

Three-Part Breath (Dirga Pranayama; sometimes called Dirga Swasam) is a gentle pranayama that is often taught to beginners because of its simplicity. As the name infers, there are three parts to this pranayama. They are the:

- abdomen

- diaphragm

- chest.

In Three-Part Breath (Dirga Pranayama), on the inhalation the breath is slowly and consciously brought into the lungs, belly, ribs, and chest. It may be helpful for your client to put one hand on their belly and one hand on the chest to see the hand on the belly expand as the breath starts there and then the hand on chest rise as the breath expands to the lungs. On the exhalation, the flow reverses, and the air leaves the chest first, then the ribs, and finally the belly.

Another way for your client to visualize the Three-Part Breath (Dirga Pranayama), if holding their hands over the chest and belly is not available to them, is to use straps for tactile feedback on the breath. One strap could be secured around the middle of the rib cage, loose enough to be snug when the client has fully inhaled, and one strap could be secured around the belly, again—loose enough so it is snug when the belly is expanded. Feeling the resistance of the strap helps clients to feel what part of their body their breath is expanding.

Precautions

This is one of the most gentle and simple pranayama. There are no precautions noted for this pranayama.

Directions

1. Instruct your client to sit comfortably on the floor (the seat or back can be supported with props), a chair with the feet resting on the floor (or blocks if the legs are not long enough to reach the floor), or other comfortable surface, including a bed if the client is not able to transfer out of the bed.

2. Instruct your client to close their eyes and place one flat hand on their belly and one on their chest (or use the strap modification noted above). Encourage them to notice their breath and not to change anything—just to notice how it feels in their body. Suggest that they stay here for approximately five breaths.

3. Encourage your client to inhale and inflate their lungs and note the air filling the belly, ribs, and chest (in that order). Encourage a pause for a moment at the top of the inhalation.

4. Instruct the client to exhale, and notice the air leaving the chest, ribs, and belly (in that order), and to notice the movement of the hands.

5. Repeat for several minutes.

Three-Part Breath (Dirga Pranayama) encourages a focus on deep and full breaths. This practice can be used at the beginning of a practice to help bring attention and centering to the individual.

Victorious Breath or Ocean Breath (Ujjayi Pranayama)

Victorious Breath or Ocean Breath (Ujjayi Pranayama) is frequently included in yoga classes, but it takes some time to get the breathing pattern down. In Ujjayi breath, the mouth is closed, and all inhalations and exhalations come from the nose. There is an audible noise associated with Ujjayi breath, which sounds like the ocean or Darth Vader, depending on your preference! To create this, the breath is constricted at the back of the throat, almost as if breathing through a thin straw. The sound is similar on the inhalations and exhalations. This practice produces heat in the body but in a gentle way. This breath is also indicated for individuals with chronic obstructive pulmonary disease (COPD), as it mimics pursed-lip breathing.

Precautions

As with other pranayama that involve breath retention (kumbhaka), caution is to be used in implementing this practice. It should not be used with individuals who have high blood pressure or heart disease. The practice should be stopped or slowed if it produces feelings of dizziness or anxiety, which may be caused by the closed mouth breathing. If this causes anxiety, encourage the client to open their mouth slightly.

Directions

1. Instruct your client to sit comfortably on the floor (the seat or back can be supported with props), a chair with the feet resting on the floor (or blocks if the legs are not long enough to reach the floor), or other comfortable surface, including a bed if the client is not able to transfer out of the bed.

2. Encourage your client to close their eyes and notice their breath. Encourage them to just notice how it feels in the body.

3. To begin, encourage your client to rest one hand on their lap and bring the other hand in front of their mouth, with their palm facing their mouth.

4. Suggest that the client inhales deeply through their nose and exhales through the mouth into the palm of the hand as if to fog up a mirror (making an audible sound on the exhale). Ask your client to repeat this several times until comfortable with these sensations, making the length of time for the inhalation and exhalation equal (Equal Breaths (Sama Vritti)). This may be enough to start with for your client. Once they feel comfortable with this, proceed to the next step.

5. Encourage the client to close their mouth and inhale deeply through their nose. Encourage them to keep their lips gently closed, exhale, and try to make the same sound as in Step 4—this sounds like the ocean or like Darth Vader. Have the client practice this for several repetitions.

6. When the client's breath is consistently audible and comfortable on the exhalation, encourage the client to focus on making the same breath sounds for both the inhalation and exhalation.

7. When these steps have been accomplished, encourage the client to practice the whole pranayama cycle for several minutes. After Ujjayi breath is mastered, it can be transferred into the physical practice, where it is paired with the physical postures.

Victorious Breath or Ocean Breath (Ujjayi Pranayama) is a versatile practice that can be used alone or in conjunction with the physical practice. However, patience is required when learning it—there are so many parts that take a while to fully understand and engage in!

Viloma Pranayama

Viloma Pranayama is a simple breathing practice to enhance relaxation. It also helps to enhance sleep, reduce anxiety, and increase lung capacity and breath control.

Precautions

This pranayama involves mild and gentle breath retention. If this causes any discomfort, encourage the client to reduce the length of time of the retention until they feel more comfortable.

Directions

1. Instruct your client to sit comfortably on the floor (the seat or back can be supported with props), a chair with the feet resting on the floor (or blocks if the legs are not long enough to reach the floor), or other comfortable surface, including a bed if the client is not able to transfer out of the bed.

2. Encourage the client to close their eyes and notice their breath for a minute.

3. Ask the client to inhale completely, feeling the belly, diaphragm, and ribs expand (as in Three-Part Breath (Dirga Pranayama)).

4. At the top of the inhalation, ask the client to concentrate on exhaling one third of their breath. Ask them to pause and then exhale another one third. Ask them to pause and then exhale the final third.

5. Encourage the client to work up to doing this for five minutes or more.

Another option for Viloma Pranayama is to pause on the inhalation or to pause on both the inhalation and exhalation. This simple pranayama can be practiced at any time.

Pranayama for Alertness
Bellows Breath (Bhastrika Pranayama)

Bellows Breath (Bhastrika Pranayama) is an activating pranayama that increases energy in the body and mind and can help with digestion.

Precautions

Caution is to be used in implementing this practice. It should not be used with individuals who have high blood pressure, heart disease, or abdominal pain. The practice should be stopped or slowed if it produces feelings of dizziness or anxiety.

Directions

1. Instruct your client to sit comfortably on the floor (the seat or back can be supported with props), a chair with the feet resting on the floor (or blocks if the legs are not long enough to reach the floor), or other comfortable surface, including a bed if the client is not able to transfer out of the bed.

2. Have your client rest their hands on the lower belly.

3. Encourage the client to close their eyes and notice their breath. Have them put their hands on their belly, with the palms open and holding their belly.

4. Ask the client to take a deep inhalation and fully expand their belly.

5. Encourage the client to forcefully exhale through the nose on the next exhalation. Then ask them to immediately inhale forcefully through the nose as fast as possible, with the long-term goal being approximately one second per cycle.

6. Encourage your client to breathe from the diaphragm and to move only their belly—not the torso or head.

7. Start with one round of this, and check in with your client to see how they feel. If they are able, continue until they have completed ten rounds.

8. After ten rounds (or sooner if needed), encourage the client to take a break and notice their natural breath cycles.

9. If possible, complete the next cycle with 20 rounds of Bellows Breath (Bhastrika Pranayama), and progress to 30 when they are ready.

Because this practice is energizing, this is a nice practice to start a therapy session or to implement if someone is feeling sluggish.

Breath of Fire or Skull Shining Breath (Kapalabhati Pranayama)

The benefits of this practice are many and include: increased internal heat; increased energy; stress reduction; increased attention; enhanced digestion; toning and strengthening of the diaphragm and abdominal muscles; and the release of toxins.

Precautions

As with Bellows Breath (Bhastrika Pranayama), caution is to be used in implementing this practice. It should not be used with individuals who have high blood pressure, heart disease, or abdominal pain. The practice should be stopped or slowed if it produces feelings of dizziness or anxiety. If this practice causes anxiety, encourage the client to open their mouth and breathe naturally through the mouth.

Directions

1. Instruct your client to sit comfortably on the floor (the seat or back can be supported with props), a chair with the feet resting on the floor (or blocks if the legs are not long enough to reach the floor), or other comfortable surface, including a bed if the client is not able to transfer out of the bed.

2. Ask your client to rest their hands on their lower belly.

3. Ask the client to close their eyes and notice their breath. Suggest that they take a deep inhale and exhale.

4. Encourage the client to inhale deeply through the nose (with their mouth closed), filling the belly until it is mostly full.

5. The goal is to quickly and forcefully exhale the air in the belly in ten short pumps of the navel towards the spine, while keeping the mouth closed. This may be very challenging, so the ten pumps can be reduced to meet the needs of your client.

6. After the last or tenth pump, encourage the client to allow their belly to fill up with air naturally with the mouth closed.

7. When the client is comfortable with this pranayama, work towards repeating Steps 4–6 up to four times.

This pranayama is a great way to start the day or a therapy session because of the energy it creates in the body. It's also a nice way to warm up on a cold day or to increase energy in the afternoon. However, this pranayama often takes a bit of practice to feel comfortable with the sensations it produces.

CHAPTER 9

Descriptions of Meditation Used in Yoga Post-Stroke

Introduction

Meditation (dhyana) is one of the essential components of a yoga practice and one of the eight limbs of yoga. However, many people feel that meditation is not for them, perhaps because they have not tried it or found a meditation practice that resonates with them. We have both heard many people say that they just can't meditate, because they can't get their brain to slow down. Buddha called this the "monkey mind," and we have both experienced this in our own minds! Meditation works to quiet the monkey mind and may take many forms, such as walking a labyrinth, something more passive and quiet, or a meditation that involves chanting mantra. No matter what form it takes, meditation is a quieting of the mind, and meditation takes practice!

Importantly, meditation may be particularly beneficial for individuals who have had a stroke. A study by Vennu and colleagues (2013) found that when 20 minutes of meditation was added to traditional stroke rehabilitation, individuals in the meditation group had greater improvements in reductions in disability, depression, and fatigue, and improved balance, compared with participants in the usual-care group, who received only conventional rehabilitation. The findings may be a result of the changes that meditation is known to make in the brain. Researchers have demonstrated that regular meditation increases the amount of gray matter in the brain—the areas that address attention, emotional regulation, and mental flexibility (Hölzel, *et al.*, 2011).

Because clients with stroke have had an insult or injury to their brain as a result of the stroke, rewiring specific pathways is essential, and meditation offers a way to do this. Therefore, suggesting regular meditation for your clients with stroke is offering them another way to increase the neuroplasticity in the brain. Meditation is also a practice that can be easily provided as homework, after instruction from the rehabilitation or yoga therapist. Meditation may also provide much-needed stress relief for the caregiver, so consider including the care provider in your instruction.

Tips for Instructing Meditation

- Most traditional forms of meditation are done seated in Easy pose (Sukhasana) on the floor; however, it can easily be modified to a chair, bed, or mat table as needed to best accommodate your clients with stroke. Because the seated meditations last for several minutes, it may be more comfortable to raise the hips by sitting on a blanket, bolster, block, pillow, or meditation cushion. In a chair, proper meditation positioning would encourage the feet to be placed firmly on the ground, with the back straight. For clients who are shorter and whose feet do not touch the ground, blocks may be used under the feet to encourage the feeling of being grounded. A sandbag can be placed on top of the feet if the client has difficulty keeping their feet on the floor. A bolster between the back and the chair (perpendicular or parallel) can also provide good support.

- Once your client is in a comfortable seated position, ensure that their spine is elongated. It is important for the client to sit with the spine as straight as possible. Ask your client to consider the visual image of the crown of the heading reaching towards the ceiling.

- The client's arms can simply rest during meditation. Encourage your client to have the hands rest in their lap or to hold them at their sides. Share with your client that it is thought that having the hands rest palms up on the knees is signaling openness, while palms down encourages grounding. Another option is to choose one of the mudras found in Chapter 10 to occupy the hands and bring added benefit during meditation.

- Cue your client to relax their shoulders. To get into the proper shoulder position, suggest that the client lifts their shoulders towards their ears, rolls the shoulder blades down the back, and lets them settle in. You can also gently place your hands on their shoulder blades and ask them to try to relax that area in response to your touch.

- Remind your client to keep their chin slightly tucked in. This should put the client's head and neck in a neutral position.

- Encourage your client to relax their jaw and mouth. This is an area where we can unknowingly hold a lot of tension.

- Ask the client to relax their gaze. During meditation, a drishti (gazing point) can provide the opportunity to focus on something in particular, or the eyes can lightly focus on something a few feet in front of the client.

- Meditation is most effective in a quiet environment. If encouraging your client to meditate, an active rehabilitation gym may not be the place to try it out. Work with your client to determine where the best location and time for a meditation may be.

- Encourage your client to make meditation a habit! The only way to reap consistent benefits from yoga is to do it every single day. Schedule a time to make meditation part of the client's daily routine.

Meditations Described

In this chapter, we offer several types of meditations. Yoga Nidra is designed to encourage a deep sleep or conscious rest. Yoga Nidra is often referred to as "yoga sleep," that is, a state of consciousness that lingers somewhere between sleep and awareness where healing of the mind and body can occur. Yoga Nidra typically lasts between 30 and 45 minutes in order to allow the mind and body time to relax into a parasympathetic state. Kirtan Kriya, from the Kundalini yoga tradition, is a meditation that involves a gazing point (drishti), and chanting (mantra). Regular practice of the Kirtan Kriya has demonstrated improvements in brain function and cognition (Black, *et al.*, 2013; Newberg, *et al.*, 2010). A walking meditation is one that focuses on the actual act of walking. Finally, mantra meditation is one that focuses on a specific mantra that is meaningful to the individual.

Yoga Nidra

Below is a Yoga Nidra script designed specifically by the authors for stroke survivors, which will last approximately 30 minutes. An audio recording may be found at www.mergingyogaandrehabilitation.com.

Directions

1. Start with the client in a supine position in a quiet environment, in their bed, on a floor, or on a mat table. If the client is not on the floor, you will need to adapt the script slightly to change "floor" to "bed" or "mat table," as appropriate. The quiet environment is key, so it is possible that the person's room in acute care may be a more therapeutic environment than the rehabilitation gym. Start by saying: "Relax fully. Keep your eyes closed. Bring your attention to the world around you. Notice the sounds outside the room. Notice the sounds within the room. Notice the sensations all around you. Notice the smells, the sounds, the temperature. Visualize your own body resting here, and focus on your heels on the floor. Notice where the back of your right leg touches the floor. Notice where the back of your left leg touches the floor. Bring your attention to your glutes, both left and right, resting on the floor. Increase your awareness to your torso, your back resting. Your left arm and fingers, resting on the floor. Your right arm and fingers, resting comfortably. The back of your head, resting on the floor or pillow."

2. The next step in Yoga Nidra is to focus on breathing. Say: "Bring awareness to your breath. Feel the breath enter your body through your nose. On your next breath, breathe into the chest and belly. Notice the breath on the exhale. On your next inhale, breathe into the left arm. Breathe into the right arm. Notice the exhale. On your next inhale, breathe into the left leg. Into the right leg. Notice the exhale. Now notice the breath on your next inhale, infusing the left arm and leg, the right arm and leg."

3. To increase awareness of the body for the next part of Yoga Nidra, say: "Bring awareness back to your body resting. Stay as still as possible. Notice your heels on the floor. Notice where the back of your right leg touches the floor. Notice where the back of your left leg touches the floor. Bring your attention to your glutes, both left and right, resting on the floor. Increase your awareness to your torso, your back resting. Your left arm and fingers, resting on the floor. Your right arm and fingers, resting comfortably. The back of your head, resting on the floor (or pillow). Sense the entirety of your whole body resting."

4. Becoming aware of bodily feeling is important. Say: "Without judgment, notice how you are feeling. Notice your emotions. Notice if your body holds any areas of tension."

5. Becoming aware of thoughts is also important. Say: "Become aware of your breath. Notice any thoughts or images that might arise as you become aware of your breath. Don't judge this, just recognize it."

6. Find joy. Say: "Think about something, a memory or a person, that brings you great joy. Stay here, imagining the way this memory makes you feel. Remember the details."

7. The final stage of Yoga Nidra is reflection. Say: "Bring awareness to your body. Become aware of your left arm, your left leg. Your right arm, your right leg. Reflect on how your body feels. Become aware of the room around you. Stretch your arms overhead, and inhale deeply. Exhale fully and bring the arms down. Come to a seated position (or have them blink their eyes open) and bring awareness back to the room."

Kirtan Kriya

Kirtan Kriya (pronounced keertun kreea) is a Kundalini meditation that involves mudras, mantra, visualization, and chanting. This meditation has been shown to: improve thinking via increased cerebral blood flow; improve memory retrieval via improved blood flow to the posterior cingulated gyrus; enhance concentration and focus via increased frontal lobe activity; enhance and increase the presence of neurotransmitters, such as norepinephrine, dopamine, and acetylcholine, which increases the functioning of the brain; lower cortisol levels, which results in increased energy levels; and improve short- and long-term psychological health and spiritual well-being (Black, *et al.*, 2013; Newberg, *et al.*, 2010). It is thought that this meditation stimulates all of the senses and the areas of the brain related to each of the senses. This meditation should ideally be done for 12 minutes, but it can be done for shorter periods of time by decreasing the minutes in relation to each other (for example, a six-minute practice would be one minute in the normal voice, one minute of whispering, two minutes of silently repeating the mantra, one minute of whispering, and one minute in the normal voice).

Directions

1. Have the client first repeat the words Saa, Taa, Naa, Maa (or mantra) while sitting with their spine straight. Often, it is helpful for individuals to understand what the words are that they are repeating in a mantra. The words Saa, Taa, Naa, Maa are considered the five primal sounds (called the panj shabd). Saying each of these words creates the cycle of creation.

   • Saa translates to infinity, cosmos, or beginning.

   • Taa translates to life, or existence.

   • Naa translates to death, change, or transformation.

   • Maa translates to rebirth.

2. The finger positions, or mudras, are very important in this meditation. Say to your client:

   i. "On Saa, touch the index fingers of each hand to your thumbs.

   ii. On Taa, touch your middle fingers to your thumbs.

   iii. On Naa, touch your ring fingers to your thumbs.

   iv. On Maa, touch your little fingers to your thumbs."

3. **Comments about these finger positions (mudras):** Each time the mudra is closed by joining the thumb with a finger, it is thought that the ego "seals" the effect of that mudra in the consciousness. According to the 3HO (2018), the name of each mudra and the associated effects are as follows:

   i. 1st finger: Gyan Mudra: Knowledge.

   ii. 2nd finger: Shuni Mudra: Wisdom, intelligence, patience.

   iii. 3rd finger: Surya Mudra: Vitality, energy of life.

   iv. 4th finger: Buddhi Mudra: Ability to communicate.

4. If the client is able to incorporate both the mantra and mudra, you can instruct the next step. Say to your client: "If possible, your focus of concentration is the L form, while your eyes are closed. With each syllable, imagine the sound flowing in through the top of your head and out through the middle of your forehead (your third eye point)."

5. The next step is to have the client repeat the mantra in three levels of volume:

   i. For two minutes, have them state the words in their normal tone of voice.

   ii. For the next two minutes, have the client repeat the words in a whisper.

   iii. For the next four minutes, have the client say the sound silently.

iv. Then reverse the order of the first two steps, whispering for two minutes and then speaking out loud for two minutes—for a total of 12 minutes.

6. To come out of the exercise, encourage the client to inhale very deeply, stretch their hands above their head, and then bring them down slowly in a sweeping motion to the lap as they exhale fully.

Walking Meditation

While this may be more challenging for someone in the earlier stages of stroke recovery, walking a labyrinth can bring great peace of mind. In the absence of a labyrinth, a walking meditation that focuses on the act of walking can be beneficial. In a walking meditation, the individual focuses on the physical sensations associated with the foot meeting the ground. Adding a mantra can increase the benefit and purposefully slow the walking. Choose something appropriate for stroke recovery, such as "I am healthy. I am whole," or choose a mantra from Chapter 5 or the sample practices in Chapter 12.

Mantra Meditation

In mantra meditation, a meaningful mantra is chosen to be repeated and focused on. Words can be self-fulfilling prophecies, and there are so many times in stroke recovery when the focus is on what the client cannot do. When instructing mantra meditation, take the time to help the client choose a positive, strength-based mantra. There are many mantras available in Chapters 5 and 12, or you can find out what is meaningful to your client. Speaking the mantra out loud also turns the meditation into a pranayama practice.

Directions

1. Ask the client to choose a comfortable position.

2. Tell them to take a few breaths and close the eyes gently.

3. Ask them to say the mantra out loud.

4. They should repeat this for several minutes.

Another way to engage in mantra meditation is to listen to an audio file that has the mantra repeating. This would be an easy way to infuse positivity into your client's stroke recovery.

CHAPTER 10

Descriptions of Mudras Used in Yoga Post-Stroke

Introduction

Mudras are hand gestures used in yoga practice that often occur in concert with meditation or pranayama and occasionally with asanas. Mudra means "seal" or "closure" in Sanskrit, and these gestures help to direct the flow of energy with the hands. Mudras are considered symbols or shapes, made with the hands, that are associated with a number of benefits, including sealing in the energy of the body.

The use of mudras is rooted in the science and practice of Ayurveda. It is believed that the different areas of the hands correspond with different areas of the brain and body so that, when a mudra is used, we are stimulating specific areas of the brain and we are creating a specific electrical/energetic circuit in the body. Thus, mudras are considered a healing modality in Ayurveda. When mudras are used in conjunction with pranayama, the prana of the body is energized. The science of Ayurveda suggests that diseases are a result of an imbalance (too much or too little) of one of the five elements: air, fire, water, earth, and space. The thumb is associated with the element of space. The index finger is associated with the element of air. The middle finger is associated with the fire element. The ring finger is associated with the element of water. The pinky finger is associated with the earth element.

The fingers act as electrical circuits and, when used in mudras, these circuits influence the flow of energy to promote health and well-being. When the fingers touch each other, they make a subtle connection, which in turn influences the subconscious reflexes in the brain. These reflexes balance and redirect the internal energy and lead to enhancements in well-being.

Mudras are very easy to use as an aspect of yoga in rehabilitation. They can be practiced in a comfortable seated position on the floor, in a chair, in bed, or on a mat table. Mudras should be practiced for at least 12 breaths and, if possible, should be coupled with Ujjayi breathing unless otherwise noted (described in detail in Chapter 8).

The practice of incorporating mudras may be challenging, because it is harder in our Western minds to understand this more ethereal view of sealing in energy as a way to promote health. Mudras are subtle, and so are the feelings associated with them. Your client (and many of us, broadly) may not feel anything while practicing a mudra, or there may be feelings of slight sensations in the hands. It may be difficult to identify the feelings or sensations as related to the mudra, and that is totally fine! There is power in the subtlety.

Using Yoga Mudras in Rehabilitation for People Who Are Post-Stroke

- While most mudras are suggested to incorporate both hands, if this is not possible because of impaired fine motor skills or hemiparesis, that is perfectly fine. Instruct the client to do the mudra with one hand and to visualize the other hand in the mudra.

- Because these mudras are subtle, it may be beneficial to talk with your client about the perceived benefits of each.

- Unless otherwise noted, it is suggested that all mudras are practiced for up to 45 minutes. This may not be possible in the rehabilitation environment or for someone who is post-stroke. Thus, it is acceptable to substantially decrease the amount of time spent practicing the mudras. Mudras also make nice, safe homework for the client to work on when not in therapy.

- In the sample intermediate practice in Chapter 12, the mudra used is simply to extend each finger and then bring each finger individually to touch the thumb. Bilateral engagement is encouraged, but this is often difficult, particularly for individuals with a hemiparetic hand. This may be a great place to start with your client, and you can then increase the diversity of mudras as dexterity improves.

The Mudras
Adi Mudra

To instruct the Adi Mudra, ask the client to have the thumb tucked into the palm, while the other four fingers wrap over it. The tip of the thumb should be reaching towards the base of the pinky finger. They can extend the hands to rest, with the palms facing down on the thighs or knees. While the client is practicing the Adi Mudra, ask them to focus on their breath. The Adi Mudra is thought to be a nice preparation for pranayama, or as a way to calm the nervous system. See Figure 10.1 for a picture of the Adi Mudra.

Benefits of the Adi Mudra include improved sleep (and reduced snoring), increased lung capacity, improved flow of oxygen to the brain, and a relaxed nervous system.

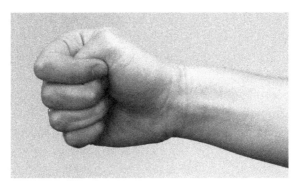

Figure 10.1

Anjali Mudra

The Anjali Mudra is widely referenced in this book and is commonly included in yoga practices. It is also called Prayer pose. To instruct this mudra, have your client bring the palms and fingers of each hand together with the thumbs towards the sternum. Ask the client to press the thumbs into the sternum lightly. Tell them to lower the chin slightly and close the eyes and then focus on the breath. See Figure 10.2 for a picture of the Anjali Mudra.

Bringing the Anjali Mudra to heart center (near the sternum) represents love and honor for the self and universe. The Anjali Mudra also helps to balance and unite the right and left sides of the body—physically, emotionally, and mentally.

The Anjali Mudra is thought to be a pathway to a meditative state and increased awareness.

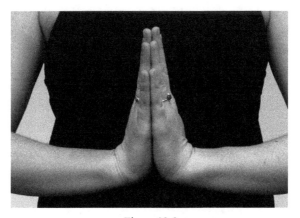

Figure 10.2

Apana Mudra

To instruct the Apana Mudra, ask the client to connect the tips of the middle and ring finger with the tip of the thumb. When the hands are in the Apana Mudra, they can rest at the sides of the body or in the lap. This mudra can be done while sitting or standing, although it is believed that greater benefits are received from doing this mudra while sitting upright. While your client is practicing this mudra, ask them to focus on their breath, noting the inhalations and exhalations. It is suggested that this mudra is practiced for 10–45 minutes, although it should not be done for two hours after a meal, because of its relationship with digestion. See Figure 10.3 for the Apana Mudra.

Apana means "downward moving force" in Sanskrit. Thus, it makes sense that the Apana Mudra is beneficial for eliminating waste from the body, as well as enhancing mental or physical digestion. The Apana Mudra helps to reduce constipation and increase regularity of bowel movements, as well as increasing urination and sweating.

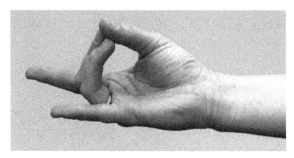

Figure 10.3

Apana Vayu Mudra

The Apana Vayu Mudra is one of the more complicated mudras. Before practicing this mudra, ask your client to rub their hands together briskly to warm them up. To instruct this mudra, ask the client to bring the tips of the middle and ring fingers to the tip of the thumb, while the pinky finger extends directly out. The index finger should be tucked near the base of the thumb. This mudra can be practiced for 15–45 minutes per day and is best practiced in a seated position. See Figure 10.4 for a picture of the Apana Vayu Mudra.

The Apana Vayu Mudra was thought to be a lifesaver from heart attacks in ancient India, and today it is thought to be beneficial for heart-related issues such as high blood pressure, palpitations, and arteriosclerosis, and for gastrointestinal issues, including heartburn and indigestion.

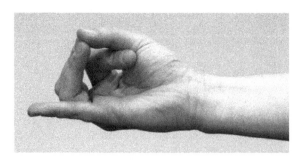

Figure 10.4

Brahma (or Purna) Mudra

For the Brahma (or Purna) Mudra, the client should be seated in an upright, comfortable position. Ask your client to create a fist with each hand and then wrap the fists around the thumbs. The knuckles for each hand are then brought to the belly and touch each other, with the palms facing upward. The client should rest their hands in this mudra in the lap, against the pubic bone. The breath should be regular and the focus simply on the inhalations and exhalations. See Figure 10.5 for a picture of the Brahma Mudra.

The benefits of the Brahma Mudra include releasing blocked energy and then releasing this energy to the brain. This mudra helps to calm the mind, enhance relaxation, and release negative energies. The Brahma Mudra is also thought to bring the individual to a higher meditative state.

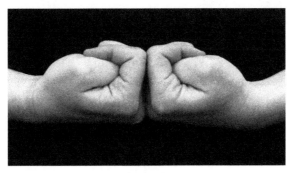

Figure 10.5

Buddhi Mudra

The tip of the pinky and the tip of the thumb press together for the Buddhi Mudra. The other fingers extend straight. Ask your client to place their hands on the thighs or knees. The focus during the Buddhi Mudra is on the normal breath cycles. See Figure 10.6 for a picture of the Buddhi Mudra.

The Buddhi Mudra enhances intuitive communication and knowledge. This mudra is thought to develop intuition, as well as provide relief from a number of ailments, including digestive issues, skin disorders, blood-related diseases, and blood and kidney disorders.

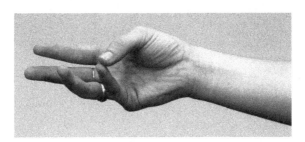

Figure 10.6

Chinmaya Mudra

To instruct the Chinmaya Mudra, ask your client to have the thumb and index finger create a circle, as in the Gyan or Chin Mudra (see Figure 10.10, further below). The other three fingers should be curled into the hand or palm. Extend the hands to rest, palms up or down, on the thighs or knees. The eyes can be closed if this is comfortable and, if possible, the breath should be in and out through the nose. This mudra can be practiced for 10–45 minutes and can be seen in Figure 10.7.

The benefits of the Chinmaya Mudra include improved digestion and enhanced flow of energy in the body, particularly in the thoracic region of the spine. The Chinmaya Mudra is also thought to promote breathing in the lungs.

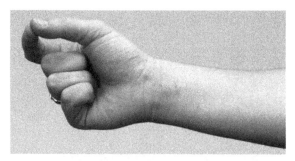

Figure 10.7

Dhyana Mudra

As mentioned earlier in this book, dhyana means meditation. The Dhyana Mudra is one to use in other meditations. It involves both hands working together—ask the client to bring the tips of each thumb together so they are touching, while the left fingers are under the palm of the right hand (which is facing up), cradling it while both hands sit in the lap. There is no specific breath focus noted in this mudra, but instruct your client to work on clearing their mind during this practice. This mudra can be seen in Figure 10.8.

In deep meditative asanas or practices, the Dhyana Mudra provides a calming energy. The Dhyana Mudra also helps to clarify thought, decreases ego involvement, and brings peace.

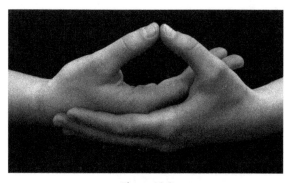

Figure 10.8

Ganesha Mudra

The Ganesha Mudra is named after the Hindu God Ganesh. Ganesh was said to remove obstacles. For this mudra, ask the client to place the left hand at sternum height in front of the chest, with the palm facing outward and the thumb facing down. The right hand should be placed in front of the left hand, with the palm open and thumb facing up. Ask the client to clasp the fingers together. In this mudra, the breath is deep and the hands are energetically pulled apart but the fingers do not separate. The client should repeat this up to six times and then reverse it so the hands switch sides. See Figure 10.9.

The Ganesha Mudra helps to remove obstacles from life and can enhance feelings of positivity and bravery in the face of difficult issues.

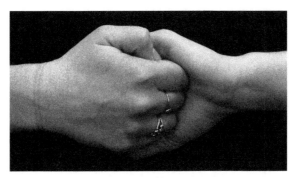

Figure 10.9

Gyan or Chin Mudra

The Gyan or Chin Mudra is similar to the OK hands position. Ask the client to have the tips of the thumb and index finger touching with the other three fingers extended as straight as possible. Tell them to extend the hands to rest, palms up, on the thighs or knees. They can note the effect of the flow of the energy in the body. The Gyan Mudra can be practiced for up to 30 minutes and its benefits may be enhanced by chanting "Om" while practicing the mudra. See Figure 10.10 for a picture of the Gyan Mudra.

Benefits associated with the Gyan Mudra include: improved concentration; stimulation of the brain and strengthening of the nervous system; increased feelings of relaxation and stress reduction; enhanced sleep; increased energy; improved focus; and reductions in lower back pain.

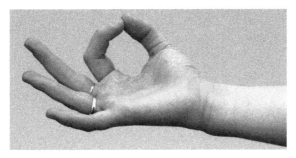

Figure 10.10

Prana Mudra

For the Prana Mudra, ask the client to bring the tips of the pinky and ring fingers to touch the tip of the thumb. The other fingers should extend straight. This is demonstrated in Figure 10.11. Note the effect of the flow of the breath (Ujjayi breathing if possible) on the body. It is suggested that the Prana Mudra should be practiced in the morning for up to 30–45 minutes.

The Prana Mudra excites and activates the energy (prana) in the body. This mudra: increases feelings of energy and strength; decreases feelings of fatigue; reduces stress; helps to improve sleep; reduces blood pressure; increases immunity; and decreases acidity and ulcers in the gut. The Prana Mudra is also thought to decrease inflammation in the body, and thus is associated with reductions in rheumatoid arthritis, and joint pain.

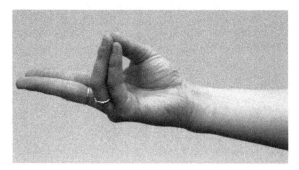

Figure 10.11

Shuni (or Shoonya) Mudra

The Shuni (or Shoonya) Mudra is much like the Gyana or Chin Mudra. Ask the client to bring the tip of the middle finger to touch the tip of the thumb and then extend the other fingers. This mudra can be done seated or standing, with the arms at the sides or resting gently in the lap. It is demonstrated in Figure 10.12.

The benefits of the Shuni Mudra include feelings of patience, discipline, and stability. The Shuni Mudra is helpful when it is difficult to complete a task and helps to bring focus and discipline.

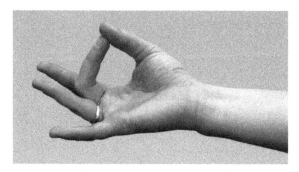

Figure 10.12

Survya Ravi Mudra

For the Survya Ravi Mudra, ask the client to bring the tip of the ring finger to touch the tip of the thumb. The other fingers should extend straight. The client's arms can rest by their side or comfortably in their lap once the mudra has been achieved. See Figure 10.13 for a picture of the Survya Ravi Mudra.

The benefits of the Survya Ravi Mudra include enhanced feelings of balance, and it brings about numerous positive changes, including physical and spiritual well-being.

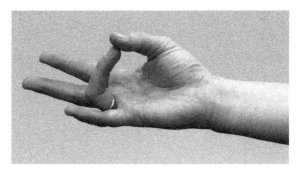

Figure 10.13

Vayu Mudra

The Vayu Mudra is similar to the Gyan or Chin Mudra. Ask the client to move the thumb so it is touching the knuckle of the index finger and exert pressure on the index finger. It is suggested that this mudra is practiced only when pain relief is needed and only for up to 10–12 minutes per day. See Figure 10.14 for a picture of the Vayu Mudra.

The Vayu Mudra is said to improve high blood pressure, abdominal discomfort, bloating, and other air-related conditions. The Vayu Mudra is also thought to improve health and decrease pain and issues from conditions including arthritis, gout, and sciatica.

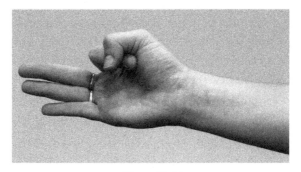

Figure 10.14

Case Reports

HOW WE AND OTHER THERAPISTS HAVE USED YOGA AFTER STROKE

We find case reports to be important teaching tools in therapy and in yoga teacher trainings. Therefore, we provide multiple case reports that include clients in different phases of their stroke recovery (including acute versus chronic, and people with varying types of post-stroke disability). We also include case reports from different types of rehabilitation therapists and one case report from us as researchers who used yoga in a study for a client with chronic stroke. These case reports include: an occupational therapist who used yoga with a client who had sustained a stroke and was being treated in the inpatient acute setting; two recreational therapists who used yoga in the acute rehabilitation setting with clients who had each sustained a stroke one month prior to treatment; and a physical therapist, who is also a yoga therapist, who treated a 22-year-old client with a recent stroke. The case reports make it clear that poses included after a stroke may vary depending on the setting, whether it is group or one-to-one therapy, and the post-stroke residual impairments of the clients. For example, the occupational therapist, Kaelyn, treated her client in a one-to-one setting and was therefore able to have her client do more complex poses, such as Downward Facing Dog (Adho Mukha Svanasana) and Happy Baby (Ananda Balasana) poses, but also prone poses, such as modified Plank (Kumbhakasana) or Cobra (Bhujangasana) poses. Such poses were not available to us in our research study where we delivered yoga in a group setting with approximately ten people per class.

These case reports are each written in the therapists' own words—thus the writing may be different from some of the other text in the book. Therapists' names are included as permitted by the therapist; however, client names are replaced with pseudonyms, unless the client specifically gave us permission to use their name. We also altered some details of the clients with pseudonyms to protect their identity. We are grateful for the therapists who have shared their stories with us and to the individuals with stroke who are included in these case reports. A special thank you to the following people:

- Leslie Willis Boslego, MS, OTR/L, RYT, who taught the yoga in our research study to groups of people with stroke, including Betty. Betty is the client's true name and is included in many of the photos in this chapter and in the book. Leslie is now an occupational therapist in southern California and is using yoga in her occupational therapy practice with veterans.

- Kaelyn Rogers, MS, OTR/L, RYT, who used yoga in addition to occupational therapy for Mary Ann who had recently sustained a stroke. Kaelyn is now an occupational therapist working in inpatient and outpatient neurorehabilitation in Boise, Idaho. Find more information about Kaelyn and her practice at www.upwardinertia.com.

- Charity Hubbard, MS, CTRS, RYT-200, who used yoga in addition to recreational therapy for Malia who had an ischemic stroke. At the time of treatment for Malia, Charity was completing her undergraduate recreational therapy internship at the Shepherd Center in Atlanta, Georgia. Charity has now graduated from the Master's program in recreational therapy at Clemson University and is using yoga in her recreational therapy practice.

- Lauren Tudor, BS, CTRS, yoga teacher, who used yoga in addition to recreational therapy for Juan, who had a cerebral artery stroke. Lauren was Charity's internship supervisor, and her primary job at the Shepherd Center is to provide yoga interventions as part of recreational therapy for inpatients and outpatients with acquired brain injury, stroke, and multiple sclerosis.

- Matthew J. Taylor, PT, PhD, C-IAYT, a yoga therapist with advanced training, who used yoga with Katie, a 22-year-old with a recent stroke. Matthew has been consistently involved with the Symposium on Yoga Therapy and Research through the International Association of Yoga Therapists. He was also the president of the International Association of Yoga Therapists (www.iayt.org) and was on its Board of Directors. You can find more information about Matthew and his practice, including his use of yoga, at http://matthewjtaylor.com.

YOGA RESEARCH STUDY
Therapist Information

Therapist name and credentials: Leslie Willis Boslego, MS, OTR/L, RYT

Background of the therapist and years of experience: At the time of the yoga research study, Leslie was a graduate student in the second year of the Colorado State University Occupational Therapy program. Arlene Schmid also attended all the yoga sessions, and Arlene is an occupational therapist with over 20 years of clinical experience and, at the time, had already run multiple yoga intervention research studies. Arlene is also a registered yoga teacher and a rehabilitation scientist who has studied movement and exercise in people with disabilities, including stroke. Arlene and Marieke (the co-authors of this book) and the research team developed the yoga intervention and Leslie delivered the intervention in a group setting. The research team included a yoga therapist involved in prior yoga and stroke studies with this team. Other research assistants were trained to provide assistance and modifications to the poses as needed.

Level of yoga teacher/therapist training: Leslie was a newly certified and registered yoga teacher (200-hour training).

Client Information

Name: Betty.

Age: 67.

Gender: Female.

Education: Some college.

Time since stroke: 7 years.

Type of stroke: Ischemic stroke.

Co-morbidities and medical history: At the time of the study, Betty self-reported that she was somewhat limited in her abilities after her stroke. She also reported multiple co-morbidities, including: high blood pressure; osteoporosis; vision impairments; hearing impairments; and pre-diabetes.

Residual impairments: Betty walked with a quad cane and sustained dense hemiparalysis to her left upper and lower extremity. Sensation and motor functioning was limited after the stroke.

Living situation: Betty lived independently in her home in the community. She also drove herself to and managed all of her own appointments.

Setting and population where this client was seen: Betty was a participant in a yoga research study. The yoga intervention took place at a university research lab in Fort Collins, CO. All participants had chronic stroke (where chronic stroke was defined as the stroke occurring longer than six months ago), so this setting would be parallel to an outpatient rehabilitation setting or a community-based yoga center.

Primary focus of yoga intervention: The yoga was delivered in a group format as part of an intervention that was focused on improving balance and balance confidence after a stroke. Previous research has shown that it is best to improve ankle and hip strength and range of motion to improve post-stroke balance. Therefore, many of the chosen physical yoga postures focused on lower extremity strength, flexibility, and balance improvement. For example, Warrior I (Virabhadrasana I) or Crescent Lunge (Anjeneyasana) may be used to stretch the hip flexors, which are often very tight after a stroke secondary to flexor contractions and prolonged amounts of time sitting. To use yoga to best improve post-stroke balance, we recommend: including balance postures, such as Tree pose (Vrksasana), Warrior I (Virabhadrasana I), or Crescent Lunge (Anjeneyasana); stretching the hip flexors with Warrior I (Virabhadrasana I) or Crescent Lunge (Anjeneyasana); increasing strength, range of motion, and proprioception through yoga practices; and improving confidence in movement and balance.

Due to the disconnect between the mind and the body that may occur after a stroke, the yoga intervention also focused on breath with movement and reconnecting the mind and body. There were research assistants available to assist with movement through postures for people with arms or legs that were hemiparetic. Therefore, as appropriate, the assistant would facilitate the movement of the arm or leg through a yoga posture, and the participants would be encouraged to watch and pay attention to the movement so that they could experience the movement and the yoga posture.

Assessment, Treatment, and Evaluation

Assessments: As this was a research study, each study participant completed many assessments before and after the eight-week yoga intervention. As the focus of the study was on balance and fall risk factor improvement, we assessed balance, balance confidence, strength, endurance, and gait speed. However, we also assessed other important issues related to post-stroke recovery, including pain and quality of life. See Table 11.1 to find out more about the assessments we included and the improvements that Betty made during the yoga intervention study.

Table 11.1: Betty's scores before and after the eight-week intervention

Assessment title	Basic assessment description	Before yoga	After yoga	Change in score as %
Berg Balance Scale	Balance test, 14 items, scores of 0–56; score <46 = fall risk. Assesses static and dynamic balance and is commonly used after a stroke (Berg, Wood-Dauphinee, and Williams, 1995).	42	54	29%
Activities Balance Confidence Scale	Balance confidence test includes 16 items, higher scores = increased confidence. Assesses confidence to maintain balance and not fall during different activities. It is commonly used after a stroke (Botner, Miller, and Eng, 2005).	55	68	24%

Assessment title	Basic assessment description	Before yoga	After yoga	Change in score as %
Sit-to-stand lower extremity strength test	Lower extremity strength test. Participant crosses arms over chest and must come to a full seat and full stand as many times as possible in 30 seconds. The sit-to-stand test is part of the Senior Fitness Test (Rikli and Jones, 2001).	9	13	44%
Bicep curl test	Upper extremity strength test. The participant completes as many full bicep curls as possible in 30 seconds (all the way down and all the way up). Men use an 8-pound weight and women use a 5-pound weight. The bicep curl test is also part of the Senior Fitness Test (Rikli and Jones, 2001).	10	15	50%
6-minute walk test	Endurance test. Participant walks as many feet as possible in six minutes. May take breaks as needed. The 6-minute walk test is also part of the Senior Fitness Test (Rikli and Jones, 2001) and is commonly used after a stroke (Pohl, et al., 2002).	677	756	12%
10-meter walk test	Gait speed (walking speed). Participants walk as fast as feels comfortable for ten meters (Perry, et al., 1995). This test is done twice and the average meters per second (m/sec) is calculated. Slow gait speed is linked to increased mortality.	.83	.91	10%
PEG test (P) pain severity, (E) enjoyment in life, (G) general activity in life	Pain interference test. Pain was assessed with the PEG, a three-item test of pain that includes average pain intensity (P), the interference of pain on enjoyment of life (E), and the interference of pain on general activity (G) (Krebs, et al., 2009). The PEG has been used with people with stroke (Miller, et al., 2013).	0	0	0
Stroke Specific Quality of Life	The Stroke Specific Quality of Life test was used to assess quality of life. It was developed by a stroke neurologist and is frequently used post-stroke. There are 12 domains and the total scores are included (Williams, et al., 1999).	250	265	6%

% change = before yoga test score – after yoga test score / before yoga test score multiplied by 100

Yoga treatment intervention: All participants in the study followed the same standardized yoga intervention. The yoga was individually adapted, as needed, to meet Betty's needs.

- **Dose of yoga—frequency, duration, intensity**:

  - Yoga was offered twice a week for eight weeks for a maximum of 16 sessions. Each session was approximately one hour long.

  - Betty attended 15 of 16 sessions.

  - In the beginning, all yoga postures were completed while sitting in a chair. During the second session, participants were told that over the next few weeks the yoga would start to become more challenging and would include standing postures and getting to the floor. Yoga became progressively more challenging over the eight weeks.

Table 11.2: Yoga poses used in the yoga research study

Seated	Standing—using a wall or a chair for support	Floor—all in a supine position or face up on a yoga mat or mat table

• Mantras
• Yoga eye exercises
• Mudras (wrist, hand, and finger movements with breath)
• Neck and head movements
• Seated flexion and Axial Extension (Rekha); lateral flexion/extension
• Spinal Twist (Jathara Parivartanasana)
• Seated Figure 4 or Pigeon (Eka Pada Rajakapotasana)
• Ankle/foot movements
• Breath work:
  – Three-Part Breath (Dirga Pranayama)
  – Victorious Breath or Ocean Breath (Ujjayi Pranayama)
  – Lion's pose (Simhasana)
  – Alternate Nostril Breathing (Nadi Shodhana Pranayama)
	• Practice with standing transfer
	• Warrior I (Virabhadrasana I)
	• Lunge or Crescent Lunge pose (Anjeneyasana)
	• Mountain pose (Tadasana)
	• Locust pose (Salabhasana)
	• Chair pose (Utkatasana)
	• Shooting Star pose (Eka Pada Utthita Tadasana)
	• Tree pose (Vrksasana)
		• Practice getting to and from the floor
		• Big Toe pose with strap as needed (Padangusthasana)
		• Bridge pose (Setu Bandha Sarvangasana)
		• Figure 4 or Pigeon (Eka Pada Rajakapotasana)
		• Anterior and Posterior Hip Tilts
		• Knees to Chest pose (Apanasana)
		• Spinal Twist to the floor (Jathara Parivartanasana)
		• Corpse pose (Savasana)
		• Mantras
		• Breath work:
		  – Three-Part Breath (Dirga Pranayama)

- **Specific postures** included in the yoga intervention study are found in Table 11.2 (additional descriptions and modifications of each asana, pranayama, and meditation can be found in Chapters 6, 8, and 9).

See Figure 11.2 for photos of Betty in Tree pose (Vrksasana) while using a chair for support. See Figure 11.2 for a photo of Betty in Warrior II (Virabhadrasana II), also using a chair for support. Because of her hemiparesis in her left arm, she is not able to raise her left arm without assistance (see Figure 11.3 for a photo of Betty receiving assistance to raise her left arm). Due to her lower extremity balance and strength, she needs to touch the chair with her right hand to help to ground her in the posture. She is not dependent on the chair to hold herself up, rather she only needs to have the chair to help her know where her body is in space. The level of assistance required will vary greatly from client to client. See Figure 11.4 for photos of Betty in supported Bridge pose (Setu Bandha Sarvangasana), with a yoga block placed under her hips. Figure 11.5 shows Betty in supine Big Toe pose (Padangusthasana), using a yoga strap to facilitate the posture. Betty reports that she continues to do Big Toe pose (Padangusthasana) on a daily basis while she is still in bed and that the pose helps to keep her lower body flexible.

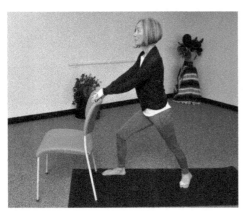

Figure 11.1

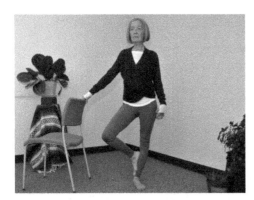

Figure 11.2

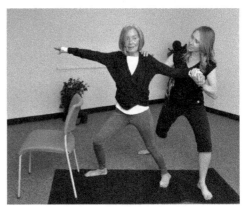

Figure 11.3

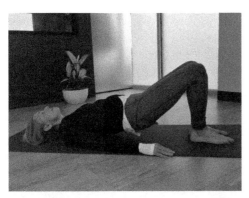
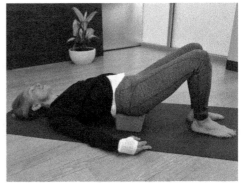

Figure 11.4

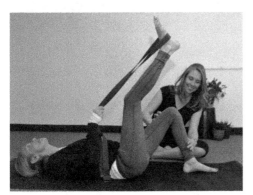
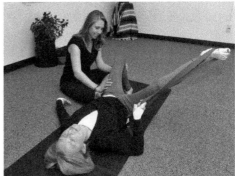

Figure 11.5

- **Breath work** was included in each session; all participants were continuously reminded to breathe and to sync each movement with the inhales and exhales, as directed. Specifically, the following were included:

  - Three-Part Breath (Dirga Pranayama), while seated in the chair and in supine. See Figure 11.6 for photos of Betty sitting in Easy pose (Sukhasana) with her hands at Prayer pose (Anjali Mudra) focusing on her breath.

  - Victorious Breath or Ocean Breath (Ujjayi Pranayama), while seated in the chair.

  - Lion's pose (Simhasana), while seated in the chair. Lion's pose (Simhasana) is a physical posture or asana. However, we place it here under breath work simply because it is placed within the yoga sequence with other breath work. Additionally, in our prior studies, the focus of Lion's pose (Simhasana) has really been on the deep inhale and the exaggerated exhale; thus participants in the study typically think of it as breath work.

  - Alternate Nostril Breathing (Nadi Shodhana Pranayama), while seated in the chair.

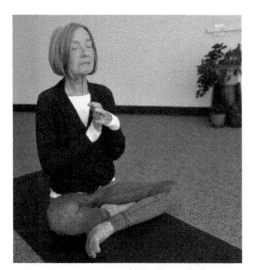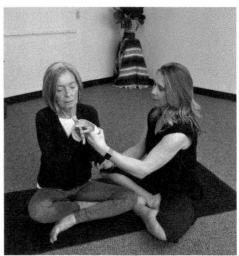

Figure 11.6

- **Mantras** were used as a way to introduce positive self-talk after a stroke and were included during each session. Mantras were stated at the beginning and the end of the practice but also during the hour-long session. Mantras included:

  - "I am enough."

  - "I am whole."

  - "I am progressing."

  - "I am loved."

  - "I am strong."

  - "I am here to do this healthy exercise. I enjoy taking time for self-care."

  - "I am taking care of myself."

- **Meditation** was included in each session and was completed while seated in the chair in the beginning of the study and while in Corpse pose (Savasana) during the later weeks of the yoga intervention. During Corpse pose (Savasana), the yoga teacher verbally directed the study participants to relax each part of their body, starting from their toes, reaching each limb, and finishing at the crown of the head. The mantra would be repeated and the participants were reminded to concentrate on their breath and the mantra. Betty can be seen in Corpse pose (Savasana) in Figure 11.7. Due to hemiparesis in Betty's left arm and leg, we simply asked that she lay comfortably in the posture. Allowing time in relaxation allowed for Betty's hand and fingers to relax; otherwise they are often held in a fist. We attempted to add a bolster under her knees, but she requested that the bolster be removed as it caused her to feel that her left knee was in an awkward position.

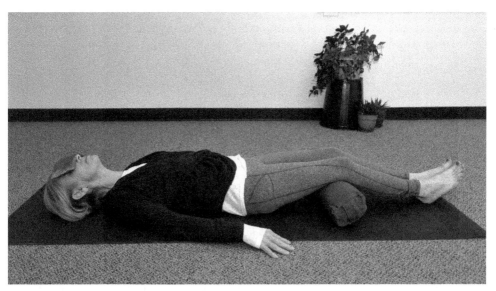

Figure 11.7

Evaluation: Betty's scores for some of her assessments are in Table 11.2. As you can see, she experienced improvements in all of these important post-stroke outcomes. In our opinion, Betty responded very well to the yoga intervention and made many comments to support this idea. For example, with practice, Betty was able to independently get to and from the floor for her yoga practice, and she commented that this made her feel much more confident in doing chores at home, as well as getting up from the floor if she did fall. On one occasion while on the floor doing postures in supine, Betty suddenly stated in a surprised voice: "I can feel my left toe again!"—and for the first time since her stroke she was able to feel her left foot, and also move her ankle through supination and pronation and dorsiflexion and plantarflexion. While this new movement made Betty feel unstable in her walking at first, with time and through yoga, she was able to strengthen the movement and she felt that the enhanced movement and sensation allowed her to improve her balance and decrease her risk of falls. Betty also reported improvements in her visual acuity, allowing her to more easily read and comprehend what she was reading. Overall, Betty reported improvements in cognitive, emotional, and physical impairments after the eight-week yoga intervention.

Two years after the study ended, Betty agreed to help us with this book and she answered some questions for us about her experience of being in the study. Below is what Betty had to say, in her own words, in response to the questions we asked of her.

Betty, you chose to be part of a research study that was merging yoga and occupational therapy for fall prevention after your stroke. We are so grateful you joined us!

- **Please tell us more about why you chose to be part of the study**: "I had participated in other Colorado State University studies. My experience was always positive. In addition, meditation or taking a few moments to clear my multitasking brain had always served me well."

- **Had you done yoga before?** "Twice."

- **Had you heard of yoga before or thought about doing yoga before?** "Yes, about eight years before my stroke. I was under extreme stress and my usual methods of compartmentalizing definitely weren't working."

- **Please talk about your experiences doing yoga with our study and team.**

  - **What did you like?** "Peaceful, safe pace which allowed for our brain delay in interpreting and attempting new or awkward actions. Addressing our brain delay early alleviated my usual frustration response which shuts down progress. Loved all the people who quietly assisted us perform the movements. Their actions allowed us to trust our bodies and our OMG I'm going to fall instincts early so we could move from protect yourself mode to I can reach or lean a little farther because my spatial touchpoint was an attentive person, not a wall or floor face plant. By the end our class, it felt like a congregation with common needs and goals. We learned a lot from each other. We confessed our fears because we trusted you would help us address them. Some of us feared falling backwards. I feared falling forward when actually there is more danger [in] leaning to my affected side. Some of the caretakers were unaware of normal stroke recovery issues such as sudden unexplained need for naps, for example. I think we all came away stronger and more knowledgeable about our new brains and bodies."

  - **What did you not like?** "I was disappointed there was not a yoga class that matched this study that I could go to after the study was over. Without the ability to continue in a safe, accessible comparable class, it's difficult not to backslide. The Seniors Yoga class is below our capacity and Beginner Yoga classes are not safe enough. (See wall/floor face plant above.)"

  - **Favorite yoga pose or part of yoga?** "I guess the eye rolls and nose pinch breathing (Alternate Nostril Breathing) under some circumstances come in handy when I am struggling to sit in a balanced posture or when my brain feels scattered. The Warrior pose helps me balance my gait and even just standing. When I over use and depend on my good side, I drag my left side along which then makes me less stable. Yoga revealed this to me and helps me remind my brain to engage the leg and foot to at least a swing instead of a drag."

– **What made the most difference to you?** "I think the whole occupational therapy with yoga was a truly holistic experience. Applying the body and real life together keeps all of it in our memory, available to pull up as needed. Important information we have to have that never occurred to us we needed. When to call an ambulance, never enter a dark room... Some of this information was obviously sitting in the dead part of our brains. I appreciate the awareness of when I'm in or out of balance and the tools to address it."

– **What were some of the benefits you remembered happening during yoga?** "I wiggled my little toe for the first time early on! By the end, I raised my affected arm over my head! I love remembering that feeling. LOL I even forget the hard work it takes to get there. Thank you for that memory."

• **Do you still do any yoga?** "I use some poses on an 'as-needed' basis when I notice slumping, sloppy gait, to ease frustration..."

  – **Why or why not?** "Tried various yoga classes, none of which met my needs. Seniors—too easy, regular—not safe. Think study wasn't long enough to instill into daily/weekly routine to reinforce doing at home alone. No accessible outside class to reinforce, even though benefits were achieved; doing yoga by oneself was not effectual without encouragement by instructor, class mates...end up just going through motions without focus."

  – **What do you need to continue with yoga?** "An actual continuing accessible specialized class. The city's current locations are a hike from parking lot to class. Too far due to thoughts of hike, I do not have the stamina to make it back to car after class."

• **What were the benefits of merging yoga with occupational therapy?** "Whole-body awareness, creating new brain memories (still remember the feeling of moving, short-circuited maybe?). We are most successful through repetition. If our daily routine doesn't include 'next steps,' we don't intuit a way to avoid danger or consider solutions. Real life shows us why prior planning is important."

- **What else do you want us to know?** "In a group someone else leads you through it. No extra multitasking involved.

"It is also the equivalent of the sense of peace received from a congregation singing the same litany and hymns. Peace, safety, reflection, taking stock, touching, looking, allowing time to recall a feeling, a movement through a visual or comment opens you to a way forward. Creating new memories and techniques helped me quell panic a lot faster if I'm caught off guard in a situation. A gift that allows me to proceed with confidence since I've relearned that I have a solution and I am capable to execute it or at least figure it out. Helped me to understand my limits. Better yet showed me pathways to an alternate solution that accommodates my disability, thanks to occupational therapy and yoga. Another bonus, I rediscovered my serenity place.

"I love this project. I feel it will really help us stroke folk have what we need as standard operating procedure. I keep thinking, 'What if I had this right after my stroke?' Now maybe others will."

YOGA DURING OCCUPATIONAL THERAPY
Therapist Information

Therapist name and credentials: Kaelyn Rogers, MS, OTR/L, RYT

Background of the therapist and years of experience: At the time that this client was seen in Virginia, Kaelyn was an occupational therapist with two years of experience.

Level of yoga teacher/therapist training: Kaelyn is also a yoga teacher and has a 200-hour teacher training with a therapeutic concentration. The training was specialized for medical professionals. As of 2018, Kaelyn had four years of experience of integrating yoga into her occupational therapy practice.

Client Information

Name: Mary Ann.

Age: 56.

Gender: Female.

Type of stroke: Brain-stem stroke with right pontine and medullary infarcts.

Co-morbidities and medical history: Obesity, diabetes mellitus, an aortic stenosis, and a previous anterior cruciate ligament injury.

Residual impairments: After her stroke, Mary Ann sustained left hemiparesis, sensory changes, impaired balance, depression, and emotional lability. She reported that she had been unable to engage in any home management tasks secondary to reduced use of the left arm, fatigue, impaired balance, and fear of falling. She demonstrated impaired range of motion in left shoulder flexion (0–130 degrees) and left shoulder abduction (0–110 degrees). At the time of her evaluation, Mary Ann's upper extremity manual muscle testing scores were below normal limits in all planes.

Living situation/discharge plan: Mary Ann lived in a townhouse with her teenage son. Her discharge plan was to return to living in the townhouse.

Setting and population where this client was seen: Mary Ann was seen for occupational and physical therapy at an acute inpatient rehabilitation center, where she also received yoga as part of an occupational therapy plan of care. Mary Ann's yoga-related goals aligned with and supported traditional physical therapy and occupational therapy. The rehabilitation center was located in central Virginia and was a state-funded rehabilitation hospital with a vocational focus.

Primary focus of yoga intervention: The yoga was delivered in a one-to-one format as part of her overall rehabilitation therapy. The primary focus of the yoga intervention was focused on education of breathing techniques, dynamic strengthening of the affected side, balance training, and trunk strengthening.

Assessment, Treatment, and Evaluation

Assessments: Clinical assessments were completed in occupational and physical therapy and included outcome measures that assessed: muscle strength (manual muscle testing); balance; endurance; mobility; activities of daily living; and instrumental activities of daily living.

Yoga treatment intervention: The yoga was individualized to meet Mary Ann's needs and focused on education of breathing techniques, dynamic strengthening of the affected or hemiparetic side, balance training, and trunk strengthening.

- **Dose of yoga—frequency, duration, intensity**:
  - Mary Ann received one-hour yoga sessions two to three times a week. Mary Ann received yoga for five weeks while attending therapy at the rehabilitation center.
  - Yoga was provided in addition to five to ten hours of traditional occupational and physical therapy provided weekly.
  - The yoga postures became progressively more challenging over the five weeks.

Table 11.3: Yoga poses used with Mary Ann and notes from her sessions

Week	Poses introduced	Movement and notes from the occupational therapist
Week 1	• Belly breathing • Mountain pose (Tadasana) • Warrior II (Virabhadrasana II) • Chair pose (Utkatasana) • Sphinx pose (Salamba Bhujangasana) • Restorative Fish pose (Matsyasana)	• All static poses. • Mountain pose (Tadasana) between each pose as a rest. • Mary Ann required a seated break every five to ten minutes. • She took more than four steps to attain a stance approximately two feet wide and required moderate assistance (mod A) to maintain balance in Warrior II (Virabhadrasana II). • She began to cry when she rolled into supine, becoming overwhelmed with excitement, as she "had not challenged [her]self to roll onto [her] stomach in 30 years." • Following this session, Mary Ann had no difficulty attaining a prone position. • During session one, Mary Ann required mod A to pull her knees into her stomach, lacking abdominal strength and stability. • With each session, she required less assistance. • A subjective comment from Mary Ann: "It just feels so great to hear that I am doing things well and to see that I can actually do this."
Week 2	• Extended Side Angle pose (Utthita Parsvakonasana) • Baby Plank pose (Kumbhakasana) • Side twists • Supported Child's pose (Balasana) • Half Frog pose (Ardha Bhekasana) • Dynamic Bridge pose (Setu Bandha Sarvangasana) • Cat Cow (Chakravakasana) • Modified Side Plank pose (Kumbhakasana) • Eagle (Garudasana)—arms only • Goddess pose (Utkata Konasana) • Half Locust pose (Salabhasana) • Happy Baby pose (Ananda Balasana)	• Mary Ann began to demonstrate increased ease and comfort. • She demonstrated an ability to step forwards and backwards up to two feet in one movement with confidence. • Decreased hands-on assistance was required, though stand-by assistance was provided. • Dynamic arm movements were introduced in order to improve the range of motion and strength in the left upper extremity. • She demonstrated an ability to move bilateral arms through all planes and sustain for up to three breaths with minimum assistance through tactile cues to achieve the full range of motion. • Mary Ann was educated on the use of myofacial release through rolling techniques; relief was reported. • She reported her pain level decreased from a 7/10 to a 0/10; no sustained increase in pain was reported for the duration of her program.

Week 3	• Downward Facing Dog (Adho Mukha Svanasana) (required support to enter and sustain) • Tree pose (Vrksasana) • Crescent Lunge pose (Anjeneyasana) • Supported Shoulder Stand pose (Salamba Sarvangasana) • Table Top (Goasana), alternating arm and leg extension • Cobra pose (Bhujangasana)	• Improved strength and fluidity. • Mary Ann demonstrated an ability to link poses together with decreased requests for breaks. • She demonstrated an ability to move the left arm through full range in all planes using the right arm to assist. • She also began to demonstrate improved overall stability and strength in the shoulder girdle and core, evidenced by ability to hold Downward Facing Dog (Adho Mukha Svanasana) with minimum assistance at the shoulder for one breath, Locust pose (Salabhasana) with arms to the side, Table Top (Goasana) with alternating arm and leg extension with contact guard assist, and Chair pose (Utkatasana) for more than ten breaths. • She demonstrated improved motor planning and body awareness, independently entering poses, aligning the body, and sustaining the posture. • During this week, Mary Ann demonstrated the ability to enter a low lunge using blocks to raise her arms. • A comment from Mary Ann during this week: "[I] often feel so weak and incompetent, and yoga makes [me] feel brave and capable."
Week	**Poses introduced**	**Movement and notes from the occupational therapist**
Week 4	• Wide Legged Forward Fold (Prasarita Padottanasana) • Wide Legged Forward Fold Twist • Warrior I (Virabhadrasana I)	During weeks 4 and 5: • Mary Ann continued to demonstrate improved strength, range of motion, motor planning abilities, and endurance. • She demonstrated an ability to ascend from and descend to the floor through a low lunge and Downward Facing Dog (Adho Mukha Svanasana) with differing levels of assistance, dependent on level of fatigue, using blocks to raise the floor and decrease workload. • Mary Ann demonstrated improved balance, beginning to try Tree pose (Vrksasana), bringing the ball of the foot to the opposite ankle with a chair at her side for support when needed. • The occupational therapist provided contact guard assist; Mary Ann maintained balance for <5 seconds on average. • A significant increase in self-confidence was noted.
Week 5	• Increased fluidity between poses and duration of each hold	

• **Specific postures** that the therapist included in the yoga intervention and the week that each was introduced are identified in Table 11.3. Notes from the occupational therapist are also included in the table. The therapeutic yoga program was designed to support occupational therapy and physical therapy goals. Yoga poses were modified as necessary, including initially eliminating transitions to and from the floor by using a raised surface, utilizing props, and modifying for decreased strength and range of motion. Hands-on assistance was provided as needed. The program was designed to continually accumulate skills, with new poses added weekly and the duration of hold increasing.

- **Breath work and mindfulness** was included in each session. Mary Ann was introduced to breathing techniques, including but not limited to Bellows Breath (Bhastrika Pranayama), Alternate Nostril Breathing (Nadi Shodhana Pranayama), and heart-opening pranayama. Initially, Mary Ann demonstrated a quick, shallow breath pattern. With continued practice, Mary Ann demonstrated independent initiation of the previously taught breathing techniques. She reported that she used these techniques in her daily life during exercise and to reduce her stress and anxiety. Mary Ann was also educated on visualization strategies and use of mantras to improve emotional regulation and overall self-confidence.

Evaluation: Multiple outcomes were assessed; however, it should be remembered that the client also received occupational and physical therapy as part of daily rehabilitation. Therefore, all changes in outcome measures are not associated with yoga. The therapist and client do, however, feel that outcomes were enhanced through the use of yoga during rehabilitation.

Regarding Mary Ann's progress, Kaelyn stated:

Continued improvement in strength was noted in the trunk and shoulder girdle, evidenced by ability to maintain positions such as Table Top (Goasana) (quadruped with opposite arm and leg extended) and modified Plank pose (Kumbhakasana) (knees dropped) for up to 45 seconds. Additionally, Mary Ann demonstrated the ability to rise from Child's pose (Balasana) through quadruped to Downward Facing Dog (Adho Mukha Svanasana) independently, and sustain Downward Facing Dog (Adho Mukha Svanasana) for up to three breaths. She demonstrated ability to move from quadruped to a low lunge without blocks to raise the chest, and found balance with shoulders flexed. She demonstrated ability to stand from a low lunge independently 75% of the time on bilateral legs, up to two times per session. Mary Ann demonstrated improved balance, evidenced by ability to maintain Tree pose (Vrksasana), without a chair for support, for up to 15 seconds on each leg, utilizing taught strategies to lengthen through the spine and standing leg. According to the physical therapy discharge report, Mary Ann scored a 56/56 on the Berg Balance test and a 24/24 on the dynamic gait index and improved her walking speed from "slow" to "slow-moderate" on the 6-minute walk test. These new skills have demonstrated carryover into her ability to independently complete home management, regaining independence in all tasks, prevocational tasks, and ability to navigate the community. Her coordination of mobility also improved (no longer requiring a cane to ambulate), and Mary Ann significantly improved her confidence in regard to balance-related activities. She demonstrated significantly improved endurance, tolerating 30–45 minutes of continuous movement without requests for a break. Finally, Mary Ann demonstrated increased upper extremity strength, as measured through manual muscle tests. Manual muscle testing is the most common way for therapists to measure strength (the results are in Table 11.4).

Table 11.4: Manual muscle testing before (baseline) and after Mary Ann completed therapy (discharge: D/C)

	Right at baseline	Right at D/C	Left at baseline	Left at D/C
Shoulder abduction	5/5	4+/5	3+/5	4/5
Shoulder adduction	5/5	5/5	4/5	4/5
Shoulder flexion	5/5	5/5	4+/5	4+/5
Shoulder extension	4/5	5/5	3/5	5/5
Elbow flexion	5/5	5/5	4/5	5/5
Elbow extension	5/5	5/5	3/5	5/5

Subjective evaluation: Mary Ann states: "Physical therapy and occupational therapy allowed [me] to increase [my] strength, but yoga increased [my] body awareness...knowing where I am in space increases my confidence so I don't feel like I'm going to tumble off." Additionally, Mary Ann attributes her participation in yoga to her decreased fear of falling, stating that she "no longer views it negatively."

Mary Ann stated that she saw the benefit of breathing exercises carry over into her physical therapy exercises and daily life—utilizing the breathing techniques taught and linking breath to movement, she began to feel an ease with movement that wasn't present before.

Mary Ann reported that yoga itself helped to motivate her. She found that yoga had the ability to "meet [me] where [I] was, and allowed [me] to better [myself] without competition." She stated that the non-competitive aspect made it fun, but she still felt as if she was constantly improving, which was encouraging and made her want to continue to engage.

Though there is no way to determine whether the same gains would have occurred without the use of therapeutic yoga, it is worthwhile to note that the client feels tremendous benefit and has stuck to the protocol for months following the cessation of inpatient treatment.

YOGA AS THERAPY DELIVERED BY A RECREATIONAL THERAPY STUDENT INTERN WHO IS ALSO A YOGA TEACHER
Therapist Information

Therapist name and credentials: Charity Hubbard, MS, CTRS, RYT–200.

Background of the therapist and years of experience: At the time of the yoga intervention, Charity was a student, completing her recreational therapy internship between her last year of undergraduate studies and the first year of a Master's degree in the Clemson University recreational therapy program in the United States. Charity was a Recreational Therapy student completing her final recreational therapy internship at the Shepherd Center in Atlanta, GA. The Shepherd Center is an internationally renowned rehabilitation center that focuses on treating clients with acquired brain injury (including stroke and traumatic brain injury), and clients with spinal cord injury. Eight weeks of Charity's recreational therapy internship was done primarily using yoga as a therapeutic intervention with Lauren Tudor's supervision. Lauren Tudor is a CTRS.

Level of yoga teacher/therapist training: Charity completed the 200-hour yoga teacher training at the Asheville Yoga Center in Asheville, North Carolina, and is a Registered Yoga Teacher through Yoga Alliance. She had taught 75 hours of yoga at the Fike Recreation Center (Clemson University's Fitness Center), 20 hours at Clemson Yoga (local studio), and 120+ hours at the Shepherd Center. Charity also trained under Lauren Tudor at the Shepherd Center to learn more therapy-focused yoga techniques, including modifications to poses and meditations designed for people with acquired brain injury or spinal cord injury.

Client Information

Name: Malia.

Age: 55.

Gender: Female.

Education: Completed high school and possibly some college.

Time since stroke: One month.

Type of stroke: Ischemic stroke.

Co-morbidities and medical history: A history of hypertension.

Residual impairments: Paralysis on the left side of her body and global aphasia.

Setting and population where this client was seen: The Shepherd Center, Atlanta, GA. The patient was seen as an inpatient on the Traumatic Brain Injury unit, in the yoga room. Note: The Shepherd Center has a yoga room on the main floor that is quiet and lit by lamps and soft candlelight. It has a different feel than most therapy spaces in an inpatient rehabilitation setting.

Primary focus of yoga intervention: The yoga was delivered in an individual format as part of a recreational therapy intervention to improve coordination, to improve balance, to decrease global aphasia symptoms, and to help reduce stress and anxiety caused from the chaotic environment of the hospital.

Assessment, Treatment, and Evaluation

Assessments: We chose a one-to-one yoga intervention and did not use any formal assessments to examine outcomes. All assessments and examinations were based on observations of the patient and any additional information given by her physical therapist. This was essentially conducted as a co-treatment with the recreational therapist and the physical therapist, who came to every yoga session. The physical therapist often gave recommendations throughout the session about what muscle groups needed to be stretched or she helped the patient move to different poses. Nearing the end of the sessions, the physical therapist participated next to Malia, while Charity taught yoga.

Planning: We did a total of four yoga sessions with Malia. The goals, from a recreational therapy perspective, were slightly different for Malia for each yoga session and included the following:

- Session 1: Develop an environment the client can feel comfortable and welcomed in. Encourage the client to express her music preferences.

- Session 2: Focus on communication and coordination, instructing the patient to move both arms at the same time.

- Session 3: Encourage the patient to learn and follow a sequence of two to three yoga moves in a row.

- Session 4: Incorporate and enhance coordination, standing, sitting, and stretching in Malia's practice.

Yoga treatment intervention

- **Dose of yoga**: Each yoga session was one hour long, and each session primarily focused on stretching and coordination. The client was encouraged to participate actively for 75% of each session, with the other 25% of the time used for meditation and relaxation.

- **Specific postures**: Mountain pose (Tadasana) (involving lifting and lowering the arms together, twisting, and standing with Malia's feet at varying distances from each other), Forward Fold (Uttanasana),

Supported Bridge pose (Setu Bandha Sarvangasana) (with a bolster under the hips), Bound Angle pose (Baddha Konasana), Seated Forward Fold (Upavistha Konasana), Child's pose (Balasana), Spinal Twist (Jathara Parivartanasana), Corpse pose (Savasana).

- **Order of postures**: Each yoga session began with standing postures and transitioned to floor postures, ending on the floor. Postures included:

  - Mountain (Tadasana)

  - Forward Fold (Uttanasana)

  - Child's pose (Balasana)

  - Seated Forward Fold (Upavistha Konasana)

  - Bound Angle pose (Baddha Konasana)

  - Supported Bridge pose (Setu Bandha Sarvangasana)

  - Spinal Twist (Jathara Parivartanasana)

  - Corpse pose (Savasana).

- **Breath work** was included in each session. We mostly used four-count Equal Breaths (Sama Vritti), each breath coming in through the nose and out through the mouth. This was in an effort to breathe with the pattern of the music and reduce the client's stress.

- **Mantras** were not included in the session. The patient was stuck in a pattern of saying "suh suh suh" and couldn't speak any other words unless they were the words to a song she knew (like Michael Jackson's "Man in the Mirror").

- **Meditation** was used throughout the session. Interoception cues were used in order to increase the client's spatial awareness. This meditation involved asking Malia to focus her attention on one body part at a time and to connect her breath with the music. The music was primarily pop music from the 1980s because Malia was more responsive and engaged when this genre was playing. Nearing the end of the intervention, traditional yoga meditation music was played to promote relaxation. There was a unique balance of engaging music to keep Malia active and calming music to help her relax.

- **Other aspects of yoga**: Malia was a unique patient in that her level of engagement was directly correlated to the song(s) playing. The yoga used had to be connected to the song playing, similar to choreography, and the songs were more upbeat than most music used in yoga. There was always a quiet, soft, and welcoming environment for her when she arrived. Blankets, straps, and bolsters were used to help her achieve the yoga poses and accommodate for left-side paralysis or increase her comfort level. Each session was very conversational; Malia moved to a pose, considered how it felt, adjusted, and moved on according to what she needed.

Evaluation: The results of this yoga intervention were very positive. The goal of increasing her coordination was achieved with the help of her physical therapist. I noticed a significant improvement in her level of energy when she came into yoga. I believe this was due to the relaxing environment. When I saw her outside of the yoga room she was often breathing rapidly and constantly scanning the room. Upon entering the yoga session, Malia began to improve her focus, which gave her an opportunity to focus on physical improvement. As she was only one month out from her stroke, her health and abilities changed daily. The improvements seen in the yoga session were more related to her general demeanor and communication. By the fourth session, Malia was able to transfer to the floor by herself, breathe evenly, and understand and follow basic instructions for yoga poses.

YOGA AS THERAPY DELIVERED BY A RECREATIONAL THERAPIST WHO IS ALSO A YOGA TEACHER
Therapist Information

Therapist name and credentials: Lauren Tudor, BS, CTRS.

Background of the therapist and years of experience: Lauren has a Bachelor's degree in Recreational Therapy from the University of Wilmington North Carolina, and at the time of the intervention Lauren had been practicing as a recreational therapist for eight years. Lauren is the yoga specialist at the Shepherd Center. She offers up to 15 classes weekly that she developed for military personnel, individuals with spinal cord injury, those with traumatic or acquired brain injury, stroke survivors, and people with multiple sclerosis. She has done specialty training with Matthew Sanford and Mind Body Solutions. She also teaches for Love Your Brain—yoga specifically for people with traumatic brain injury. Lauren is actively working to increase involvement with research on yoga with traumatic brain injury through the Shepherd Center. She is close to completing her advanced yoga therapy training (500 hours) through the Center for Integrative Yoga Studies and is in the process of becoming a certified yoga therapist (C-IAYT).

Level of yoga teacher/therapist training: Lauren completed a 200-hour yoga teacher training from Pranakriya in Atlanta, GA, along with extensive other trainings, including adapted yoga certification levels 1 and 2 with Mind Body Solutions and Love Your Brain yoga teacher training certification, and is close to completing her 500-hour yoga teacher training from the Center for Integrative Yoga Studies.

Client Information

Name: Juan.

Age: 38.

Gender: Male.

Education: College (level and number of years were unspecified).

Time since stroke: One month.

Type of stroke: Left middle cerebral artery stroke.

Residual impairments: Right-sided weakness, aphasia.

Setting and population where this client was seen: Juan was seen during inpatient rehabilitation at the Shepherd Center, Atlanta, GA, on the Acquired Brain Injury unit. Yoga was delivered as part of therapy, in conjunction with physical, occupational, recreational, and speech therapy.

Primary focus of yoga intervention: To help the client to reengage in a previous interest, increase relaxation, improve range of motion, engage in stretching, increase body and breath awareness, improve attention to task, and improve communication.

Assessment, Treatment, and Evaluation

Assessments: Relaxation, mood, body awareness, and range of motion.

Planning: Juan's goals included a return to his previous interests, knowledge of relaxation techniques, increasing body awareness, and reducing aphasia.

Yoga treatment intervention

- **Dose of yoga—frequency, duration, intensity**: Yoga sessions were held one time per week, for one hour per session, and for a total of seven weeks.

- **Specific postures** included the following:

  - Weeks 1–3: All postures were done in supine position on the floor.

  - Weeks 3–5: We began on the floor in supine position and then moved to seated yoga postures. No standing postures were utilized during this timeframe.

  - Weeks 5–7: We began in standing position, moved to seated position, and then to supine position.

- **Order of postures**:

  - Weeks 1–3: Legs over a bolster to begin with breathing and relaxation (Corpse pose (Savasana) with a bolster under the knees), Bridge (Setu Bandha Sarvangasana), arm stretch and reach, Figure 4 leg stretch (also known as Supine Pigeon) (Supta Eka Pada Rajakapotasana), Reclining Hand to Big Toe pose (Supta Padangusthasana) with assistance and yoga strap, Reclining Twist (Jathara Parivartanasana), Modified Fish pose (Matsyasana) with a bolster, Body Scan Meditation focused on interoception, Corpse pose (Savasana).

  - Weeks 3–5 in supine: Legs over a bolster to begin with breathing and relaxation (Corpse pose (Savasana) with a bolster under the knees), Bridge (Setu Bandha Sarvangasana), arm stretch and reach, Figure 4 (also known as Supine Pigeon) (Supta Eka Pada Rajakapotasana), Reclining Hand to Big Toe pose (Supta Padangusthasana) with assistance and yoga strap, Reclining Twist (Jathara Parivartanasana), Modified Fish pose (Matsyasana) with a bolster, Seated Mountain pose (Tadasana), Cat Cow (Chakravakasana), neck stretch, seated twist, seated meditation, Corpse pose (Savasana).

  - Weeks 5–7: Mountain pose (Tadasana) with a focus on balance and breath, Mountain pose (Tadasana) with arm flow, Downward Facing Dog (Adho Mukha Svanasana) with hands on elevated mat, Forward Fold (Uttanasana), folding forward towards an elevated mat table for support, seated Cat Cow (Chakravakasana), Bridge pose (Setu Bandha Sarvangasana), Spinal Twist (Jathara Parivartanasana), Corpse pose (Savasana).

Breath work was used in each session. This was primarily Three-Part Breath (Dirga Pranayama) and some Victorious Breath or Ocean Breath (Ujjayi Pranayama).

Mantras were not used during this yoga intervention.

Meditation was used during the intervention. The meditation techniques that were used included guided body scanning, relaxation, and progressive muscle relaxation.

Evaluation: Juan responded well to yoga sessions and said that he enjoyed coming to class. He progressed well during his inpatient rehabilitation stay. During Week 1, Juan needed maximum assistance to get on and off the floor, maximum assistance with all right-side movements and postures, and intermittent assistance for improved comfort positioning. He appeared to be holding a significant amount of tension throughout his body and he did not speak or make eye contact. I noticed improvements weekly during our yoga sessions. By the fourth session, Juan could transfer to the floor and move into different positions with minimal assistance and was able to understand and follow directions for yoga poses and pranayama. I also noticed changes in Juan's mood and confidence. He started greeting me with a smile and making eye contact with me. I noticed that he was less guarded with his movements and his posture improved. I believe he was more relaxed as his communication and body awareness continued to improve and he could understand the breathing techniques. By the last session, Juan was having short conversations with me and laughing at jokes. He thanked me for the yoga sessions and was inquiring about continuing yoga in his outpatient program.

YOGA AS THERAPY DELIVERED BY A PHYSICAL THERAPIST WHO IS ALSO A YOGA THERAPIST
Therapist Information

Therapist name and credentials: Matthew J. Taylor, PT, PhD, C-IAYT.

Background of the therapist and years of experience: At the time, Matthew was a 57-year-old male, and he was a 1981 US Army/Baylor Master's of Physical Therapy graduate. Matthew, at the time, had 20 years of yoga therapy experience and had completed his PhD in 2005. The focus of his doctoral research was on a yoga school for chronic spine pain. He then opened and ran a yoga-based rehabilitation clinic (using no conventional rehab equipment), Dynamic Systems Rehabilitation PLLC, in Scottsdale, AZ, from April 2004 through May 2016, where this patient was seen. Presently, Matthew is not seeing patients; he is instead using his time writing books, teaching yoga in rehab online, and still leading professional development within yoga therapy and the International Association of Yoga Therapists (www.iayt.org).

Level of yoga teacher/therapist training: Matthew has extensive training in yoga, with over 2000 hours of training in yoga teaching and yoga therapy. Additionally, his doctoral work was focused on yoga. He initiated the standards and accreditation process within the yoga therapy profession, and he is a liaison between the International Association of Yoga Therapists and licensed healthcare providers, working to set policy and professional relationships.

Client Information

Name: Katie.

Age: 22.

Gender: Female.

Education: Finishing undergraduate studies in journalism at a high-profile university.

Time since stroke: Six months.

Type of stroke: Left subarachnoid hemorrhage secondary to anatomical anomaly.

Residual impairments: Mild to moderate right hemiparesis with spasticity in dominant right upper extremity and weakness in right lower extremity. She wore an ankle foot orthosis on the right lower extremity and used a straight cane on uneven surfaces and terrains. Handwriting and keyboarding was slow and awkward for Katie, due to motor control impairments after the stroke.

Living situation: Katie lived independently at her school during the semester and at home with her parents otherwise. She was a senior journalism student at a major university and had a semester remaining prior to graduation. She wasn't cleared for driving yet and managed all her own appointments, with her father supporting her through driving her to attend the appointments.

Setting and population where this client was seen: Katie was seen at the above-noted clinic, in Scottsdale, AZ. She was young and still completing her college education when she had a stroke. Katie was undergoing conventional rehabilitation at the major university hospital system while at school and was going through conventional rehabilitation at the Valley's premier stroke center while on her break from school. Staff therapists there had recommended consultation and treatment at Dynamic Systems Rehabilitation to incorporate additional mind and body psychosocial interventions. In addition to her rehabilitation, she'd been undergoing a series of Botox injections to decrease right upper extremity spasticity.

Primary focus of yoga intervention: The primary focus of the yoga therapy intervention was to establish a supportive, compassionate, self-aware, mind-body practice that Katie could adapt and enhance across her lifetime. This treatment intervention was grounded in expanding her appreciation for the web of relationships her lived experience and lived body were immersed in, to include her current rehabilitation, career aspirations, and personal life. The stroke permanently altered her self-identity and that hadn't yet been addressed deeply, and certainly not from an embodied exploration to include her relationship with self (niyamas) and others (yamas). The exploration too of "right work" given her new identity was central in order for Katie to have meaning and purpose contextually tied to a life well lived, rather than her striving to be "normal" in a non-normal experience and all the consequent suffering tied to overcoming the impacts of the stroke versus acceptance and adapting. At its basic core, right work surrounds the ethics of earning a living and may be also known as right livelihood in Buddha's pathway.

Assessment, Treatment, and Evaluation

See Table 11.5 for a general outline of therapy and treatment strategy. We utilized: pranayama; mudra; audible mantra (integration of glottal/upper thoracic sensing and control from vocalization and also a postural control model for standing stability and upper extremity platform); and focal asana, including attention to sensing and moving and a remapping of both sensory and motor maps (including synching movement with breath, attending to various sensations, and regularly shifting attention within the same therapeutic exercise pattern, i.e. feet, breath, face, floor, etc.). Therapy included homework to read yamas and niyamas and to apply them to her life situation. Also, reading assignments around right work and Ayurveda were included. Regular Yoga Nidra was included to practice withdrawal of reaction to sensation (both somatic and thinking-as-sensation). Katie recorded the Yoga Nidra sessions on her phone (see Chapter 9 for a Yoga Nidra practice). The therapist also introduced the use of slow-motion recording on Katie's phone and she recorded her gait and upper extremity movements. This allowed her to bring in awareness visually, fully sensing the "whole" versus a hyper-focus on the specific moment or movement.

Assessments: See goals and outcomes in Table 11.5.

Table 11.5: Challenges, goals, and outcomes for Katie

Challenge	Goal	Outcome
Sympathetic breathing pattern with elevated shoulders, clenched abdomen, and visible upper quarter accessory respiratory muscles.	Increase awareness of the pattern, provide strategies for shifting to diaphragmatic breathing, and softer accessory tone.	Katie was able to sense breath pattern and use postural support/attention and conscious recruitment to quiet the central nervous system for improved movement performance.
Katie was bored with the upper-extremity, fine-motor, home exercise program and often skipped her exercises.	Expand understanding of necessary sensation/motor planning/feedback loop and how to create multiple variations to prior rote motions.	Katie could demonstrate the goal and shared system with conventional rehab team, especially sensing the motor action at the location of the muscle versus "staring" at her fingertips wanting them to move differently. She was regularly performing and refining her fine-motor home exercise program.

Fear/sympathetic override and chest breathing with gait training challenges.	Bring attention down into her pelvis and lower extremities, while softening chest breathing pattern, sensing and accepting support (asana principles) versus gripping and bracing in drills.	Katie was much more at ease, especially in lateral and retro drills as well as over destabilized surfaces and with visibility-reduced environments. Noted increased confidence in activities of daily living and engagement in more challenging surfaces for greater freedom of movement.
No awareness of relationship of lower body to upper body in both gait and upper extremity function	Discover relationship through postural stability and control how each area informs the other, so when facing a challenge, she has options beyond just "trying harder" and would look to extended relationships for support or modification to enhance performance.	She could verbalize the relationships and list additional strategies beyond trying harder for both gait challenges and upper extremity movements.
Daunted by career goals given her new lived body reality after the stroke.	Explore yamas and niyamas, as well as Ayurvedic "right work" options, and edit her personal narrative to generate eased and optimized motor function platform (versus underlying stress or fear foundation).	She had numerous options to explore, and had been reading voraciously on systems, ecology, and motor control theory, as well as mind-body medicine; discovering a niche both excited her but was also "hot" as a topic to sell.
Heavy "thinker" without much embodied awareness historically. Tended to override sensory input to achieve goals by efforting.	Develop daily embodied practice to bring balance to efforts and goals, keeping a sense of self-compassion and humor versus strict, judgmental attitude to her experiences.	In addition to her embodied home exercise program, she also went to bed with a Yoga Nidra practice every night, noting enhanced sleep pattern and being quicker to chuckle at her own deeply engrained efforting habit.

Planning: The goals of the yoga therapy sessions were to respond to Katie's recent challenges of that day or the day prior. In addition to optimizing her overall autonomic nervous system state, we wanted to model and instruct her in how to create new responses to what, after six months, was feeling like fixed patterns of frustration or goal blocking. We began and ended each session with centering and setting our intentions (sankalpa) for the practice and for the day. Our focus included short-term, immediate goals, but also her longer-range vocational concerns. We frequently reviewed her home exercise program from her conventional rehabilitation provider as material to convert or augment with mind-body tweaks. Katie found this helpful, and she reinforced the idea at the next visit with the original rehabilitation therapist who had originally recommended that Katie try yoga therapy with Matthew.

Yoga treatment intervention

- **Dose of yoga—frequency, duration, intensity**: Matthew stated: "Little is known regarding dosing of yoga, so we use what we know from neuroplasticity rehabilitation studies, including importance of salience, frequent and many repetitions." Matthew included a big emphasis on using activities of daily living as "off-the-mat" yoga throughout the day.

- **Specific postures**: Simple, functionally related, grounding through the feet, extremity alignment, sensing into the pelvis, and softening the throat and neck...over and over.

- **Order of postures**: Start with sensing/centering/relaxation postures, then build out onto quieted system. Varied from sitting, supine, and standing to mimic everyday life.

- **Breath work**: Opening/releasing the throat and collarbones/armpits, keeping the face and eyes soft (to manage all that "over striving habit"). Generally Cooling Breath (Sitali Pranayama) was also included in the practice (langhana).

- **Mantras**: Both audible and internal mantras were included with Katie. Beja mantras for interoceptive training and awareness were included and were complemented by mudras for the chakras. All mantras and mudras focused on attention to the thalamic sensory and motor map refreshment. Beja mantras are used to expand and widen one's mind using the power of sound vibration.

- **Meditation**: Given Katie's busy, thought-chasing mind, Matthew included the use of Yoga Nidra to generate a meditative state versus having Katie trying to meditate.

- **Other aspects of yoga**: Yamas, niyamas, and Ayurveda were addressed and were focused on her development of a new self-identity and her future career decisions.

Evaluation: Matthew saw Katie four times over a six-week break from school, at which time she was returning for her final semester.

- **Were goals met?** All of the goals were "in progress," given the short period of the therapeutic intervention. See the goals in Table 11.5 for additional details.

- **Subjective comments**: Katie was enthused to explore her professional goals and future vocation in light of her experience of having a stroke.

She was also considering how she could leverage her unique lived experience to find a niche in the very competitive journalism market, plus have her work support her rehabilitation. She stated that this eased her prior worries over livelihood, etc. She also noted that the mindful asana-like qualities she learned to bring to her exercises relieved much of the tedium and frustration she'd been experiencing before yoga therapy. Of particular interest to her was discovering the systems connection between her injury and her love of ecological science and environmental studies that she wanted to focus her future writing toward.

- **Did the client respond well?** Yes; as her mood became more stabilized, she found that having the embodied practices readily available to her was directly impactful when she was under stress. This was increasingly a true comfort to her and also helped to improve her sense of efficacy. She also noted increased confidence when approaching challenging terrains, such as new learning opportunities (awkward asana-like) versus fear of failure or just exercises in frustration.

- **Were there any unexpected (positive or negative) outcomes?** Many of the above experiences were unexpected on her part, but not from Matthew's clinical perspective. Katie seemed to also appreciate how the yoga therapy visits were purposely responsive to her immediate experiences and insights, specific to her living with her condition, and specific to her day or week since the last visit. This is in comparison to more traditional therapy that may follow a pre-established schedule of goals that may or may not have been applicable during that visit. The sense of co-creating in the moment had the dual benefit of being even more of a participant intervention (her other programs were top notch, so this isn't a knock on them), but, also, she got to experience how to use the techniques to address real-time challenges and to not be dependent on an outside expert to apply responses to her present circumstances. This valuing of her lived experience gave her hope that she was better prepared to "live with" her new body and the new mind-body relationship as an ongoing creative process, versus a ball and chain to drag along with her for the rest of her life.

There was not any long-term follow up, as the clinic closed during her last semester away at school.

CHAPTER 12

Sample Yoga Practices

Sequences for One-to-One, Group, and Restorative Practices for Acute and Chronic Stroke

In this chapter, we introduce sample practices that the yoga or rehabilitation therapist may use with clients with stroke. Many of the yoga asanas, pranayama, mudras, and meditations included here are fully described in Chapters 6–10. In addition to the descriptions of the practices, we incorporate helpful modifications for the poses, including chair modifications when possible. A list of the benefits associated with some of the more common poses are found in Chapter 13.

Below we include both one-to-one practices and group practices to allow for flexibility. Following those, we include two sample restorative yoga practices to enhance relaxation and stress relief and soothe the nervous system for clients with stroke. Practices in the one-to-one yoga sessions are typically more challenging and should only be completed once the therapist is comfortable with the client's current level of function, as well as the therapist's ability to modify postures and maintain safety during the therapeutic session. Restorative practices can be used in acute or chronic stroke for any level of functioning.

For each sample yoga practice or session, we include:

- important notes related to the session

- goals for the yoga session that the yoga or rehabilitation therapist may consider using to address their client's needs. These are a mix of goals that the yoga or the rehabilitation therapist may consider for a client or for the session in general (and they may be the goals of the therapist)

- mantras to consider for the session

- a list of postures and breath work to include in the session. A resting meditation is included at the end of each practice

- a hand out for the therapist that includes drawings of each yoga pose to enhance the delivery of the yoga intervention.

These practices should be modified to best meet the needs of the client with stroke, and their caregiver, as appropriate.

The perceived benefits of many of the identified yoga poses or breath work are found in Chapter 13. Reasons to include the postures or breath work are based on both clinical reasoning as therapists and our knowledge as yoga teachers, including the knowledge of the yoga teachers and therapists who helped to develop the yoga and deliver the interventions used in our research studies. Some of this information is based on the science of yoga therapy; however, as there is little science supporting these details, much of the information is based on our yoga teacher trainings and the literature that surrounds yoga.

This is not a fully comprehensive list, as there is little research in regard to the benefits of specific yoga poses and because often the benefits of yoga seem to be from the whole practice, not just certain postures that are included in a practice. But in including our reasoning and the perceived benefits of the poses we chose to include in the sample practices, we hope to assist the therapist in choosing the best and most therapeutic yoga poses and breath-work practices for their clients with stroke.

Yoga During the Acute Phases of Stroke (Inpatient Rehabilitation)

Inpatient rehabilitation is where many occupational, recreational, physical, and/or speech therapists work with clients who have recently sustained a new stroke. We previously completed a research study where we added yoga to ongoing therapies at an inpatient rehabilitation facility (Schmid, *et al.*, 2015b; Van Puymbroeck, *et al.*, 2015). All study participants received their normal and prescribed occupational, recreational, physical, and/or speech therapies. In addition to traditional therapies, individuals were invited to also choose to attend yoga sessions. Yoga was offered in group and one-to-one sessions and all yoga was taught by a yoga therapist (Nancy Schalk). Group yoga was offered twice a week for 45-minute-long sessions. The one-to-one sessions were also offered twice a week but for 30 minutes. The one-to-one sessions were sometimes at the bedside but were also completed in other areas of the hospital, including the outdoor garden or therapy gym. A few individuals chose to engage in both group and one-to-one sessions of yoga, allowing up to four sessions of yoga a week. Because study participants were in the early phases of recovery, were receiving hours of therapy a week, and were admitted to an inpatient rehabilitation facility, most, if not all, clients would show great improvements regardless of yoga.

Our purpose was to determine whether patients would choose to do yoga, whether therapists would recommend yoga, and whether yoga seemed beneficial to add to ongoing inpatient rehabilitation. It appears that the answer to all of our questions was—yes! The majority of individuals invited to attend yoga agreed to attend and 97% of the study participants recommended yoga to others during inpatient rehabilitation. We found that therapists were happy to refer clients to receive yoga during the inpatient stay, as the therapists thought that the yoga would be beneficial to different clients, including those with stroke. Overall, individuals who received yoga thought that yoga helped their breathing, relaxation, and psychological well-being. Additionally, the individuals in the study were satisfied with the yoga program but would have liked yoga to be offered more frequently.

Below we provide a sample of a yoga practice that could be delivered in a one-to-one setting as well as a group setting. In the acute setting, it is more likely that the therapist is integrating yoga into some other aspect of rehabilitation and is likely not able to provide as many poses or an hour of yoga. However, we know that more and more rehabilitation facilities are in fact providing yoga in addition to traditional therapies—therefore we provide a longer yoga session, and the therapist may modify the practice as necessary.

The handouts featured in Chapters 12 and 13 can be downloaded to print from www.jkp.com/voucher using the code XEOKYDY.

ONE-TO-ONE YOGA SESSION IN THE ACUTE SETTING

Session Notes

- Clients with a new stroke in the acute setting are at great risk for falls or other health complications. Safety is paramount for this population.

- In order to stay in the inpatient rehabilitation setting, clients are required to attend many hours of occupational, recreational, physical, and/or speech therapy a day and to make progress in their recovery.

- During the stay in this setting, it is common for the client to require many other tests to assess recovery and other medical complications (consider MRI, blood work, etc.). These tests may be the cause of great anxiety and worry—the test itself may be scary, but the outcome may be scarier.

- People who have recently sustained a stroke are often in shock that they had a stroke and are still very upset that the stroke occurred.

- Clients with new stroke will likely process cues and information slowly, so use as few words as possible to direct movement and give them time to follow instruction. It is likely the client will need tactile cues and time to be successful in completing postures and breath work.

- During the acute phase of recovery, it is recommended that the client does not complete any type of inversion where the head would be below the heart. For example, the therapist should not attempt to have the client complete Downward Facing Dog (Adho Mukha Svanasana) while in prone (on the floor face down) but could consider Downward Facing Dog (Adho Mukha Svanasana) at the wall. See Chapter 6 for descriptions and modifications of poses. We include Downward Facing Dog (Adho Mukha Svanasana) (at the wall) in this sample practice; note that this may be too much for many clients with an acute stroke, but, if possible, do consider it.

- Yoga poses in prone may be considered, but only if the therapist and the client feel comfortable with moving into these poses. It may be helpful to use a mat table rather than the floor when going into prone positions. There are good reasons for moving into quadruped and other postures that include all limbs touching the ground; for example, being in quadruped or Table Top (Goasana):

  - is considered therapeutic and is commonly used in therapy

  - helps with asymmetry, which is common after stroke

  - gives proprioceptive feedback into the limb/limbs that has/have hemiparesis

  - is grounding to the client.

- Use a gait belt/transfer belt as needed to move from sitting to standing or to transfer to the floor.

- This sample yoga practice includes sitting, standing, and floor postures. Sitting yoga postures may be completed while the client is at the edge of the bed, on a mat table, or in a chair. If the practice is to be completed while sitting in a chair, please note the following points:

  - Chairs should *not* have wheels.

  - We recommend using chairs with arms to help clients feel more secure; the arms provide some leverage for different yoga postures and movements.

  - Some clients (particularly clients who are shorter) may require a block under each foot so they are not swinging their legs; this helps the client to feel more grounded in their practice and less distracted.

Possible Goals

- Help the client realize that they can control their own breath.

- Teach the client to use their breath to manage stress and anxiety during rehabilitation and other necessary medical procedures.

- Help the client to learn to integrate yoga into daily recovery.

- Help the client to use yoga, breath work, and meditation to be in the present moment and focus on their recovery and their future and to stop ruminating about the recent stroke or the losses since the stroke.

Mantras

In this setting, the client will have sustained the stroke very recently; therefore the therapist may want to consider the following mantras: "I am whole," "I am alive and I am grateful," or "I am enough."

Postures and Breath Work

Each posture is completed with the inhale and the exhale; if comfortable, postures may be held for two to three breaths. Postures, breath work, and meditation are presented here in the order that each is to be completed, but this may be modified by the yoga or rehabilitation therapist as necessary.

- Seated:
  1. Centering with the eyes closed, *state the mantra for today's session.*
  2. Take notice of the breath:
     i.   Three-Part Breath (Dirga Pranayama)
     ii. extended exhale
     iii. *repeat the mantra.*
  3. Alternate Nostril Breathing (Nadi Shodhana Pranayama).
  4. Lateral neck flexion to each side.
  5. Neck flexion.
  6. Axial Extension (Rekha).
  7. Hand to opposite knee for a slight rotation or twist and crossing the midline.
  8. Seated Forward Fold (Upavistha Konasana) (only if not concerned about falling out of the chair).
  9. Breath of Fire/Skull Shining Breath (Kapalabhati Pranayama).

- Standing:
  1. Come to standing.
  2. For support in standing use:
     – the back of a chair for support as needed
     – the wall
     – the therapist
     – nothing, if this is appropriate and safe.
  3. Mountain pose (Tadasana).
  4. Shoulder rolls, forward and backward.
  5. Mountain pose (Tadasana).

6. Lateral side flexion to each side, one arm up towards the ceiling and the other arm down towards the ground, with axial spinal extension for the transition from one side to the other.

7. Mountain pose (Tadasana).

8. Toe/ball of foot lifts, little lifts/bounces.

9. Leg extension (one-legged, modified Locust pose (Salabhasana)), left leg back.

10. Warrior I (Virabhadrasana I), left leg back.

11. Mountain pose (Tadasana).

12. Downward Facing Dog (Adho Mukha Svanasana) with assist and done at the wall.

13. Leg extension (one-legged, modified Locust pose (Salabhasana)), right leg back.

14. Warrior I (Virabhadrasana I), right leg back.

15. Mountain pose (Tadasana).

16. *Repeat the mantra.*

Transfer to the floor for floor postures in both prone (face and belly towards the floor) and supine (face up):

- Prone poses:

   1. Quadruped or Table Top (Goasana).

   2. Cat Cow (Chakravakasana).

   3. Quadruped or Table Top (Goasana).

   4. Look towards left hip or c-curve, look over left shoulder.

   5. Quadruped or Table Top (Goasana).

   6. Look towards right hip or c-curve, look over right shoulder.

   7. Quadruped or Table Top (Goasana).

   8. Child's pose (Balasana).

   9. Roll to supine with assist.

- Supine poses:

  1. Knees to Chest (Apanasana).

  2. Bridge pose (Setu Bandha Sarvangasana).

  3. Supine on floor with knees bent, resting pose.

  4. Figure 4 or Pigeon (Eka Pada Rajakapotasana), left leg.

  5. Ankle/foot movements, left leg.

  6. Knees to Chest (Apanasana).

  7. Figure 4 or Pigeon (Eka Pada Rajakapotasana), right leg.

  8. Ankle/foot movements, right leg.

  9. Bridge pose (Setu Bandha Sarvangasana).

  10. Knees to Chest (Apanasana) or simply hug the knees.

  11. Supine on floor with knees bent, resting pose.

  12. Big Toe pose (Padangusthasana), using yoga strap or gait belt, left leg to the ceiling, left leg into abduction.

  13. Transition yoga or gait belt to the other leg.

  14. Big Toe pose (Padangusthasana), using yoga strap or gait belt, right leg to the ceiling, right leg into abduction.

- Final relaxation and meditation:

  1. Corpse pose (Savasana) with eye pillow.

  2. Three-Part Breath (Dirga Pranayama).

  3. *Repeat the mantra.*

  4. Progressive relaxation, going from the toes to the crown of the head, bringing a focus to each body part and then letting it go.

HAND OUT 12.1: ONE-TO-ONE YOGA SESSION IN THE ACUTE SETTING ☑

Follow the sequence from left to right of each row. Start from a seated position.

Seated postures	Center breath work (mantra)	Alternate Nostril Breathing (Nadi Shodhana Pranayama) (mantra)	Lateral neck flexion to each side
Neck flexion	Axial Extension (Rekha)	Spinal Twist (Jathara Parivartanasana), left and right	Seated Forward Fold (Upavistha Konasana)
Breath of Fire/ Skull Shining Breath (Kapalabhati Pranayama)	**Standing postures**	Mountain pose (Tadasana)	Shoulder rolls, forward and backward
Mountain pose (Tadasana)	Lateral side flexion to each side	Mountain pose (Tadasana)	Toe/ball of foot lifts, little lifts/bounces
Leg extension, left leg back	Warrior I (Virabhadrasana I), left leg back	Mountain pose (Tadasana)	Downward Facing Dog (Adho Mukha Svanasana) at the wall

Leg extension, right leg back	Warrior I (Virabhadrasana I), right leg back	Mountain pose (Tadasana) (mantra)	**Prone floor postures**
Quadruped or Table Top (Goasana)	Cat Cow (Chakravakasana)	Quadruped or Table Top (Goasana)	Look over or c-curve to left
Quadruped or Table Top (Goasana)	Look over or c-curve to right	Quadruped or Table Top (Goasana)	Child's pose (Balasana)
Roll to supine with assist	**Supine floor postures**	Knees to Chest (Apanasana)	Bridge pose (Setu Bandha Sarvangasana)
Supine on floor, knees bent, resting pose	Figure 4 or Pigeon (Eka Pada Rajakapotasana), left leg	Ankle/foot movements, left leg	Knees to Chest (Apanasana)
Figure 4 or Pigeon (Eka Pada Rajakapotasana), right leg	Ankle/foot movements, right leg	Bridge pose (Setu Bandha Sarvangasana)	Knees to Chest (Apanasana) or simply hug the knees

Supine on floor, knees bent, resting pose	Big Toe pose (Padangusthasana) and left leg into abduction	Big Toe pose (Padangusthasana) and right leg into abduction	Corpse pose (Savasana) (mantra)
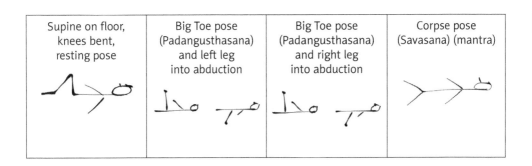			

GROUP YOGA SESSION IN THE ACUTE SETTING

Session Notes

- Review and consider the important session notes for the One-to-One Yoga Session in the Acute Setting.

- Consider whether your group session in the acute setting includes only clients with stroke or other people with disabilities, and adjust the group and the practice accordingly. Our research indicates that people with different disabilities (i.e. stroke, multiple sclerosis, traumatic brain injury, chronic pain) can successfully be integrated into a yoga group session together. It is also possible to teach yoga in a group with only clients who have sustained a stroke. Either way, a mixed group or a group of just clients with stroke is feasible and beneficial, but it appears there are pros and cons to both.

- Safety is paramount, as the individuals in the group will have all had a recent stroke. Most yoga poses in a group setting for people with an acute stroke should likely be sitting. People may sit on mat tables in the therapy gym, in their wheelchairs (with the brakes locked), or in other chairs that have arms and do *not* have wheels.

- When practicing in a group in the acute setting, we recommend only including standing poses if the therapist feels comfortable and confident with the clients moving from sitting to standing. The entire practice may be completed in sitting and still be very beneficial to the group of clients. See Chapter 6 for descriptions and modifications of each pose.

- If the therapist includes standing postures, make sure that clients who wish to remain sitting know they can continue while seated and can still be successful and benefit from the seated practice. The therapist should know all of the seated modifications for each standing pose to use as necessary. Review chair modifications in Chapter 6.

- Have clients use the chairs or the wall for standing postures when in a group, regardless of their ability to stand independently (unless there are other assistants or therapists around to assist and prevent a fall or injury).

Possible Goals

- Consider using goals from the One-to-One Yoga Session in the Acute Setting.

- As this is a group session, consider a goal regarding:

  - appropriate social interactions, if that is an issue for the clients

  - communication issues related to aphasia or dysarthria, for example a goal may be for the "client to speak at least one time to another group member."

Mantras

This may be the first time that clients are interacting with new people since the stroke occurred. They may be concerned about how they look or how they sound. Consider mantras such as "We are here and we are enough," "We are here together, and together we will progress," "We feel good today," or "We are stronger together."

Postures and Breath Work

Each posture is completed with the inhale and the exhale; if comfortable, postures may be held for two to three breaths. Postures, breath work, and meditation are presented here in the order that each is to be completed, but this may be modified by the yoga or rehabilitation therapist as necessary.

- Seated:

  1. Centering with eyes closed, *state the mantra for today's session.*

  2. Take notice of the breath:

     i.   Three-Part Breath (Dirga Pranayama)

     ii. extended exhale

     iii. *repeat the mantra.*

  3. Alternate Nostril Breathing (Nadi Shodhana Pranayama).

  4. Lateral neck flexion to each side.

  5. Neck flexion.

  6. Axial Extension (Rekha).

  7. Eye exercises, including focusing on a drishti (gazing point).

8. Seated Cat Cow (Chakravakasana).

9. Seated Forward Fold (Upavistha Konasana) (only if not concerned about falling out of the chair).

10. Lion's pose (Simhasana).

11. Seated Spinal Twist (Jathara Parivartanasana) to both sides, arms up towards the ceiling, and axial spinal extension for the transition from one side to the other.

12. Seated Forward Fold (Upavistha Konasana) (only if not concerned about falling out of the chair).

13. Lateral side flexion to each side, one arm up towards the ceiling and the other arm down towards the ground, with axial spinal extension for the transition from one side to the other.

14. Seated Forward Fold (Upavistha Konasana) (only if not concerned about falling out of the chair).

15. Seated Figure 4 or Pigeon (Eka Pada Rajakapotasana), left leg.

16. Ankle/foot movements, left foot.

17. Seated Forward Fold (Upavistha Konasana) (only if not concerned about falling out of the chair).

18. Seated Figure 4 or Pigeon (Eka Pada Rajakapotasana), right leg.

19. Ankle/foot movements, right foot.

20. Seated Forward Fold (Upavistha Konasana) (only if not concerned about falling out of the chair).

- Standing:

  1. Come to standing, move behind the chair, and hold on to the back of the chair for support (remind the client it is perfectly fine to do all of these postures in sitting as well; review the chair modifications in Chapter 6).

  2. Mountain pose (Tadasana).

  3. Shoulder rolls, forward and backward.

  4. Shoulders to ears.

  5. Shoulders down the back.

  6. Mountain pose (Tadasana).

  7. Leg extension (one-legged, modified Locust pose (Salabhasana)), left leg back.

8. Crescent Lunge pose (Anjeneyasana), left leg back.

9. Warrior I (Virabhadrasana I), left leg back.

10. *Repeat the mantra.*

11. Mountain pose (Tadasana).

12. Shooting Star (Eka Pada Utthita Tadasana), left leg out.

13. Mountain pose (Tadasana).

14. Five Pointed Star (Utthita Tadasana).

15. Leg extension (one-legged, modified Locust pose (Salabhasana)), right leg back.

16. Crescent Lunge pose (Anjeneyasana), right leg back.

17. Warrior I (Virabhadrasana I), right leg back.

18. *Repeat the mantra.*

19. Mountain pose (Tadasana).

20. Shooting Star (Eka Pada Utthita Tadasana), right leg out.

21. Five Pointed Star (Utthita Tadasana).

22. Mountain pose (Tadasana).

- Seated:

  - Final relaxation and meditation:

  1. Rub the hands together to generate warmth.

  2. Place the hands over the eyes and nose.

  3. The hands may stay on the face or in the lap for the relaxation.

  4. *Repeat the mantra.*

  5. Progressive relaxation, going from the toes to the crown of the head, bringing a focus to each body part and then letting it go.

HAND OUT 12.2: GROUP YOGA SESSION IN THE ACUTE SETTING ☑

Follow the sequence from left to right of each row. Start from a seated position.

Seated postures	Center breath work (mantra)	Alternate Nostril Breathing (Nadi Shodhana Pranayama) (mantra)	Lateral neck flexion to each side
Neck flexion	Axial Extension (Rekha)	Eye exercises	Cat Cow (Chakravakasana)
Seated Forward Fold (Upavistha Konasana)	Lion's pose (Simhasana)	Spinal Twist (Jathara Parivartanasana) left and right	Seated Forward Fold (Upavistha Konasana)
Lateral side flexion left and right	Seated Forward Fold (Upavistha Konasana)	Figure 4 or Pigeon (Eka Pada Rajakapotasana), left leg	Ankle/foot movements, left leg
Seated Forward Fold (Upavistha Konasana)	Figure 4 or Pigeon (Eka Pada Rajakapotasana), right leg	Ankle/foot movements, right leg	Seated Forward Fold (Upavistha Konasana)

Standing postures	Mountain pose (Tadasana)	Shoulder rolls, forward and backward	Shoulders to ears
Shoulders down the back	Mountain pose (Tadasana)	Leg extension, left leg back	Crescent Lunge pose (Anjeneyasana), left leg back
Warrior I (Virabhadrasana I), left leg back, mantra	Mountain pose (Tadasana)	Shooting Star (Eka Pada Utthita Tadasana), left leg out	Mountain pose (Tadasana)
Five Pointed Star (Utthita Tadasana)	Leg extension, right leg back	Crescent Lunge pose (Anjeneyasana), right leg back	Warrior I (Virabhadrasana I), right leg back
Mountain pose (Tadasana)	Shooting Star (Eka Pada Utthita Tadasana), right leg out	Five Pointed Star (Utthita Tadasana)	Mountain pose (Tadasana)
Seated postures	Seated Corpse pose (Savasana) (mantra)		

Yoga During the Chronic Phases of Stroke

Typically, individuals who sustained their stroke more than six months ago are considered to be in the chronic phases of stroke recovery. Due to neuroplasticity, discussed in Chapter 2, cognitive, emotional, and physical changes are still very possible during the chronic phases of stroke. With eight weeks of yoga, we have seen substantial improvements in people with stroke, even as much as 20 or 30 years after the occurrence of the stroke. Our studies have included people in their late 80s and early 90s, who demonstrated that improvement is possible and likely with yoga.

ONE-TO-ONE YOGA SESSION IN A SETTING FOR CLIENTS WITH CHRONIC STROKE

When providing yoga as therapy in a one-to-one setting, the yoga or rehabilitation therapist may be able to provide much more challenging poses and pranayama for the client than in a group setting. The therapist has to decide whether they are integrating yoga into the hour of occupational, recreational, physical, and/or speech therapies, or if the entire session will be a yoga practice, potentially delivered by the yoga therapist. The occupational, recreational, physical, and/or speech therapist likely has to address goals based in their discipline, and yoga may be a modality or a piece of the intervention puzzle. For others, yoga is fully the intervention. These factors will greatly influence the yoga provided in a one-to-one setting and may be dependent on the setting and other important factors. Below, we provide a sample of a full yoga practice—lasting approximately 90 to 120 minutes—but the therapist is encouraged to include what is necessary, basing their choices of postures and breath work on the benefits of the poses or the goals of the session and the client.

Session Notes

- All notes from the acute sessions are important to review; however, the chronic stroke population does have different needs.

- As this is a yoga practice for a one-to-one setting and for a client with a chronic stroke (at least six months post-stroke), the sample includes seated, standing, and floor postures, and is overall more challenging than other sample practices provided elsewhere in this chapter.

- It is thought that, in the acute setting, if the client's blood pressure is high or unstable, the head should not be below the heart. However, because we are more comfortable with inversions for people with chronic stroke, we therefore include Downward Facing Dog (Adho Mukha Svanasana) as a yoga pose to consider. This should, of course, only be done if the therapist is confident and competent in assisting the client through the pose, and if the client is ready (physiologically and emotionally) for the pose. Downward Facing Dog (Adho Mukha Svanasana) may be completed at the wall if a safe modification is needed.

Possible Goals

- Improve standing and sitting posture.

- Improve balance and reduce falls.

- Improve endurance.

- Help the client to use their breath to calm their mind and body.

- Integrate yoga into daily recovery.

Mantras

As this client will have sustained the stroke at least six months ago, they are in the phase of chronic stroke recovery. Here the client may be wondering if there is still room for recovery but may need help knowing they are exactly where they should be right now. Consider using the mantras of: "I am enough," "I am whole," or "I am taking care of my mind and my body."

Postures and Breath Work

This is the most challenging of the included sample practices and will take approximately 90 to 120 minutes. The therapist should be comfortable modifying poses or the order of poses to best meet the needs of the client. Each posture is completed with the inhale and the exhale; if comfortable, postures may be held for two to three breaths. Postures, breath work, and meditation are presented here in the order that each is to be completed, but this may be modified by the yoga or rehabilitation therapist as necessary.

- Seated (in a chair, or more advanced clients may begin the practice on the floor or a mat table):

    1. Centering with eyes closed, *state the mantra for today's session*.

    2. Take notice of the breath:

        i.   Three-Part Breath (Dirga Pranayama)

        ii. extended exhale

        iii. *repeat the mantra.*

    3. Alternate Nostril Breathing (Nadi Shodhana Pranayama).

    4. Mudras (wrist, hand, and finger movements with breath).

    5. Lateral neck flexion to each side.

    6. Neck flexion.

7. Axial Extension (Rekha).

8. Eye exercises.

9. Seated Forward Fold (Upavistha Konasana) (only if not concerned about falling out of the chair).

- Standing:

1. Come to standing and move behind the chair.

2. For support in standing use:

   – the back of the chair for support as needed

   – the wall

   – nothing, if this is appropriate and safe.

3. Mountain pose (Tadasana).

4. Shoulder rolls, forward and backward.

5. Mountain pose (Tadasana).

6. Breath of Fire/Skull Shining Breath (Kapalabhati Pranayama) (do while sitting if not safe in standing) or Lion's pose (Simhasana) while standing and holding on to the chair.

7. Lateral side flexion to each side, one arm up towards the ceiling and the other arm down towards the ground, with axial spinal extension for the transition from one side to the other.

8. Mountain pose (Tadasana).

9. Leg extension (one-legged, modified Locust pose (Salabhasana)), left leg back.

10. Warrior I (Virabhadrasana I), left leg back.

11. Warrior II (Virabhadrasana II), left leg back.

12. Extended Side Angle (Utthita Parsvakonasana), left leg back.

13. Mountain pose (Tadasana).

14. Chair pose (Utkatasana).

15. Mountain pose (Tadasana).

16. Leg extension (one-legged, modified Locust pose (Salabhasana)), right leg back.

17. Warrior I (Virabhadrasana I), right leg back.

18. Warrior II (Virabhadrasana II), right leg back.

19. Extended Side Angle (Utthita Parsvakonasana), right leg back.

20. Mountain pose (Tadasana).

21. Five Pointed Star (Utthita Tadasana).

22. Shooting Star (Eka Pada Utthita Tadasana), left leg out.

23. Shooting Star (Eka Pada Utthita Tadasana), right leg out.

24. Mountain pose (Tadasana).

25. Chair pose (Utkatasana).

26. *Repeat the mantra.*

27. Mountain pose (Tadasana).

28. Tree pose (Vrksasana), including focusing on a drishti (gazing point), left leg grounded and right foot up.

29. Mountain pose (Tadasana).

30. Tree pose (Vrksasana), including focusing on a drishti (gazing point), right leg grounded and left foot up.

Transfer to the floor for floor postures in both prone (face and belly towards the floor) and supine (face up):

- Prone poses:

    1. Quadruped or Table Top (Goasana).

    2. Cat Cow (Chakravakasana).

    3. Quadruped or Table Top (Goasana).

    4. Downward Facing Dog (Adho Mukha Svanasana)—if the therapist and client feel ready.

    5. Quadruped or Table Top (Goasana).

    6. Child's pose (Balasana).

    7. Prone Locust pose (Salabhasana), pose for two or three repetitions.

    8. Cobra pose (Bhujangasana) or Sphinx pose (Salamba Bhujangasana).

    9. Child's pose (Balasana).

    10. Roll to supine with assist as needed.

- Supine poses:

  1. Knees to Chest (Apanasana).

  2. Head turns to left and right with arms out to the side in cactus arms.

  3. Bridge pose (Setu Bandha Sarvangasana).

  4. Anterior and Posterior Hip Tilts.

  5. Bridge pose (Setu Bandha Sarvangasana).

  6. Supine on floor with knees bent, resting pose.

  7. Figure 4 or Pigeon (Eka Pada Rajakapotasana), left leg.

  8. Ankle/foot movements, left leg.

  9. Knees to Chest (Apanasana).

  10. Figure 4 or Pigeon (Eka Pada Rajakapotasana), right leg.

  11. Ankle/foot movements, right leg.

  12. Bridge pose (Setu Bandha Sarvangasana).

  13. Supine on floor with knees bent, resting pose.

  14. Spinal Twists (Jathara Parivartanasana) with knees bent, to both the left and the right.

  15. Knees to Chest (Apanasana) or simply hug the knees.

  16. Windshield Wiper Legs.

  17. Big Toe pose (Padangusthasana), using yoga strap or gait belt, left leg to the ceiling, left leg into abduction.

  18. Big Toe pose (Padangusthasana), using yoga strap or gait belt, right leg to the ceiling, right leg into abduction.

  19. Supine on floor with knees bent, resting pose.

  20. Happy Baby pose (Ananda Balasana).

- Final relaxation and meditation:

  1. Corpse pose (Savasana) with eye pillow.

  2. Three-Part Breath (Dirga Pranayama).

  3. *Repeat the mantra.*

  4. Progressive relaxation, going from the toes to the crown of the head, bringing a focus to each body part and then letting it go.

HAND OUT 12.3: ONE-TO-ONE YOGA SESSION IN A SETTING FOR CLIENTS WITH CHRONIC STROKE

Follow the sequence from left to right of each row. Start from a seated position.

	Center breath work (mantra)	Alternate Nostril Breathing (Nadi Shodhana Pranayama) (mantra)	Mudras
Seated			
Lateral neck flexion to each side	Neck flexion	Axial Extension (Rekha)	Eye exercises
Seated Forward Fold (Upavistha Konasana)	**Standing postures**	Mountain pose (Tadasana)	Shoulder rolls, forward and backward
Mountain pose (Tadasana)	**Supine floor postures**	Bridge pose (Setu Bandha Sarvangasana)	Supine on floor, knees bent, resting pose
Figure 4 or Pigeon (Eka Pada Rajakapotasana), left leg	Ankle/foot movements, left leg	Knees to Chest (Apanasana)	Figure 4 or Pigeon (Eka Pada Rajakapotasana), right leg
Ankle/foot movements, right leg	Bridge pose (Setu Bandha Sarvangasana)	Supine on floor, knees bent, resting pose	Spinal Twist (Jathara Parivartanasana), knees bent, left, right

Knees to Chest (Apanasana) or simply hug the knees	Breath of Fire/ Skull Shining Breath (Kapalabhati Pranayama)	Lateral side flexion to each side	Mountain pose (Tadasana)
Leg extension, left leg back	Warrior I (Virabhadrasana I), left leg back	Warrior II (Virabhadrasana II), left leg back	Extended Side Angle (Utthita Parsvakonasana), left leg back
Mountain pose (Tadasana)	Chair pose (Utkatasana)	Mountain pose (Tadasana)	Leg extension, right leg back
Warrior I (Virabhadrasana I), right leg back	Warrior II (Virabhadrasana II), right leg back	Big Toe pose (Padangusthasana), abduction, left	Big Toe pose (Padangusthasana), abduction, right
Supine on floor, knees bent, resting pose	Happy Baby pose (Ananda Balasana)	Corpse pose (Savasana) (mantra)	Extended Side Angle (Utthita Parsvakonasana), right leg back

Mountain pose (Tadasana)	Five Pointed Star (Utthita Tadasana)	Shooting Star (Eka Pada Utthita Tadasana), left leg out	Shooting Star (Eka Pada Utthita Tadasana), right leg out
Mountain pose (Tadasana)	Chair pose (Utkatasana) (mantra)	Mountain pose (Tadasana)	Tree pose (Vrksasana), right foot up
Mountain pose (Tadasana)	Tree pose (Vrksasana), left foot up	**Prone floor postures**	Quadruped or Table Top (Goasana)
Cat Cow (Chakravakasana)	Quadruped or Table Top (Goasana)	Downward Facing Dog (Adho Mukha Svanasana)	Quadruped or Table Top (Goasana)
Child's pose (Balasana)	Locust pose (Salabhasana)	Cobra (Bhujangasana) or Sphinx pose	Child's pose (Balasana)

Supine floor postures	Knees to Chest (Apanasana)	Cactus arms and head turns	Bridge pose (Setu Bandha Sarvangasana)
	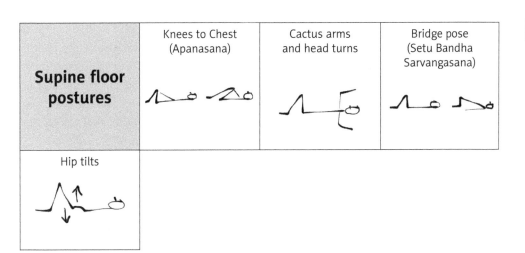		
Hip tilts			

Group Yoga Session in a Setting for Clients with Chronic Stroke

The sample yoga practices in this section may be appropriate for people with a chronic stroke (longer than six months after the stroke occurred), and therefore might be used in outpatient rehabilitation or in a group or community-based setting. We include three separate yoga practices that could be used in a group setting. These practices are derived from our research studies where we offered group yoga twice a week for eight weeks (16 sessions) (Schmid, *et al.*, 2012). Here we include a beginning practice (all in sitting), an intermediate practice (sitting and standing), and a more advanced practice (for Week 7 or 8, and including sitting, standing, and supine/floor postures). Detailed descriptions and modifications of the poses, breath work, meditations, and mudras may be found in Chapters 6–10. Here, we include a list of poses, breath work, mantras, and meditations to be considered for an hour-long group yoga session for a beginner, intermediate, and more advanced practice for clients with chronic stroke.

BEGINNING GROUP PRACTICE: ALL IN SITTING (SESSION 2 OF 16)

Session Notes

- All notes from the One-to-One Yoga Session in a Setting for Clients with Chronic Stroke are important to review.

- This beginning practice was used for the first week of the research study and was developed so that all individuals felt successful in their yoga postures. All postures were completed in sitting and assistants were available to help clients move limbs into postures, follow instructions, and identify the left from the right limb.

- During this session, we let clients know that they would soon begin to complete yoga postures while standing and that they may use the chair or the wall to maintain balance and safety. We also let them know that they would begin to get to the floor in a few weeks to complete yoga postures on the floor (in supine). We let them know that some of the most beneficial postures for them would be best done on the floor while laying down on their backs...and that Corpse pose (Savasana) is much more relaxing and comfortable while lying on their backs. Clients with stroke are often nervous about getting to the floor; they are worried about falling or not being able to get back up. We have found that introducing future floor poses during Session 2 helps to alleviate some worries about getting to the floor during the future yoga sessions, starting in Week 5 (Session 9). This early introduction to the idea of moving to the floor allows us to build relationships so that clients trust us. We also give clients enough time and warning, so that they begin to feel more confident and comfortable in their own body and with their abilities. Additionally, in hospitals and other rehabilitation settings, clients may wish to be able to use a fold-down mat table rather than get to the floor. With assistance, all of the individuals in our research studies have been able to safely and successfully get to and from the floor. However, some clients do prefer to use a fold-down mat table or to remain sitting and not go to the floor. As therapists who are using yoga after stroke, we strive to treat the client as an individual, meeting them where they are and helping them to meet their individual needs. As we are teaching the clients to honor their own mind and body, we allow them to make their own decisions about moving to the floor for their yoga practices.

- During each session, we provided yoga blocks and yoga straps to be used for modifications as necessary.

- This entire practice is to be completed while sitting in a chair.

  - Chairs should *not* have wheels.

  - We recommend using chairs with arms to help clients feel more secure; the arms provide some leverage for different yoga postures and movements.

  - Some clients may require a block under each foot so they are not swinging their legs; this helps the client to feel more grounded in their practice and less distracted.

- As necessary, it is important to provide tactile and verbal cueing through this session to remind clients to sit up straight. Tactile cueing involves the therapist placing one hand on the client's intermediate to upper back and slightly pushing towards the heart and placing the other hand on the front of the client's shoulder and slightly pushing towards the heart. With these tactile and verbal reminders, we have typically seen an improvement in sitting and then standing posture by Week 3 of an eight-week intervention. See Figure 12.1 of the therapist

(Arlene) providing tactile cueing to Betty to improve her posture. As needed, the therapist may use the same placement of hands to enhance posture while in standing.

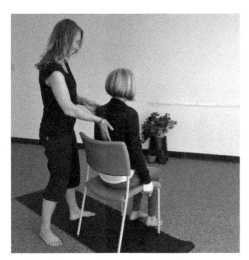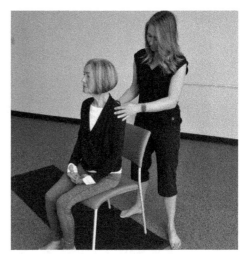

Figure 12.1

Possible Goals

- Begin to address the mind and body connection through breath work.

- Use tactile and verbal cueing to remind the client to sit up straight.

- Ensure that the client feels successful in their yoga practice.

Mantras

This is the first group yoga class and for some clients it may be a new experience to be surrounded by other people with stroke. Consider using a mantra, such as "We are here, we are taking care of our minds and our bodies," "We are here together to care for ourselves," "Be here now," "We are here now," or "Together we will progress."

Postures and Breath Work

Each posture is completed with the inhale and the exhale; if comfortable, postures may be held for three to five breaths. Seated postures, breath work, and meditation are presented here in the order that each is to be completed, but this may be modified by the yoga or rehabilitation therapist as necessary.

1. Centering with eyes closed, *state the mantra for today's session.*

2. Take notice of the breath:

    i.   Three-Part Breath (Dirga Pranayama)

    ii.   extended exhale

    iii.   Victorious Breath or Ocean Breath (Ujjayi Pranayama)

    iv.   *Repeat the mantra.*

3. Eye exercises, including focusing on a drishti (gazing point).

4. Seated Cat Cow (Chakravakasana).

5. Shoulder rolls, forward and backward.

6. Shoulders to ears.

7. Shoulders down the back.

8. Lateral neck flexion to each side.

9. Neck flexion.

10. Axial Extension (Rekha).

11. Cactus arms, arms back to lap, repeat.

12. Lateral side flexion to each side, may use the chair arm for assistance, one arm up towards the ceiling and the other arm down towards the ground, with axial spinal extension for the transition from one side to the other.

13. Eagle (Garudasana)—arms only.

14. Seated Forward Fold (Upavistha Konasana) (only if not concerned about falling out of the chair).

15. Seated Figure 4 or Pigeon (Eka Pada Rajakapotasana), left leg.

16. Ankle/foot movements, left foot.

17. Seated Figure 4 or Pigeon (Eka Pada Rajakapotasana), right leg.

18. Ankle/foot movements, right foot.

19. Seated Spinal Twist (Jathara Parivartanasana) to both sides, arms up towards the ceiling, and axial spinal extension for the transition from one side to the other.

20. Seated Forward Fold (Upavistha Konasana) (only if not concerned about falling out of the chair).

– Final relaxation and meditation:

1. Rub the hands together to generate warmth.

2. Essential oils may be used if desired (check allergies).

3. Place the hands over the eyes and nose.

4. The hands may stay on the face or in the lap for the relaxation.

5. *Repeat the mantra.*

6. Progressive relaxation, going from the toes to the crown of the head, bringing a focus to each body part and then letting it go.

HAND OUT 12.4: GROUP YOGA SESSION IN
CHRONIC STROKE: BEGINNING

Follow the sequence from left to right of each row. Start from a seated position.

Seated postures	Center breath work (mantra)
Eye exercises	Cat Cow (Chakravakasana)
Shoulder rolls, forward and back	Shoulders to ears
Shoulders down the back	Lateral neck flexion, left and right
Neck flexion	Axial Extension (Rekha)
Cactus arms x 2	Lateral side flexion, left and right

Eagle (Garudasana)—arms only	Seated Forward Fold (Upavistha Konasana)
Figure 4 or Pigeon (Eka Pada Rajakapotasana), left leg	Ankle/foot movements, left foot
Figure 4 or Pigeon (Eka Pada Rajakapotasana), right leg	Ankle/foot movements, right foot
Spinal Twist (Jathara Parivartanasana), left and right	Seated Forward Fold (Upavistha Konasana)
Seated Corpse pose (Savasana) (mantra)	

INTERMEDIATE PRACTICE WITH STANDING POSTURES (SESSION 8 OF 16)

Session Notes

- All notes from the One-to-One Yoga Session in a Setting for Clients with Chronic Stroke and the Beginning Group Practice: All in Sitting (Session 2 of 16) are important to review.

- Each session builds on the prior session; therefore, some postures and breath work are the same each week and other postures become more advanced over the eight weeks.

- Yoga Session 8 includes both sitting and standing postures. Clients were invited to begin standing postures during Session 3, so clients have had a lot of needed practice by Session 8.

- Standing postures can be modified through the use of the back of the chair or the wall. With time, some clients will become more independent in their standing postures and will no longer need the physical modifications. On some days, some individuals may need to choose to complete the standing poses while in sitting (see Chapter 6 for pose modifications).

- Mountain pose (Tadasana) is commonly used in transitions from one pose to the next pose during the standing postures. While Mountain pose (Tadasana) is most commonly completed with the arms down to the side, the arms may also be up in extension over the head, depending on the needs and the abilities of the clients. Having the arms over the head may lead to fatigue or may not be possible with an arm that is hemiparetic.

- There are quite a few poses included in this session. We purposefully increase the number of poses to increase the challenge of the yoga practice. Additionally, as clients gain confidence and skill, they are able to move in and out of each posture more quickly. Depending on the clients and the setting, the therapist may need to alter this practice by decreasing or increasing the number of planned poses during the session.

- Always ask that clients listen and honor their bodies. If they feel unstable or as if standing is not a good idea, invite the client to sit for all or part of the practice.

- Forward folding may decrease blood pressure and may lead to dizziness for some clients. Moving from sitting to standing may also lead to dizziness due to changes with blood pressure (orthostatic hypotension). Make sure clients are reminded that dizziness may occur for numerous reasons and that they should remain sitting, or sit down, if they become dizzy for any reason. Give another reminder for the client to listen to their own body.

- This is the last session before we begin to include floor postures during Session 9. Due to clients' concerns and worries about not being able to get up from the floor or about getting down to the floor, we remind them of how exciting it will be for them to progress their yoga practice by getting to the floor. We also remind them of how much stronger and more flexible they were than just a few weeks ago.

- Continue to provide cueing regarding sitting and standing posture, but by Session 8 it is likely that you just have to tap the person or give a verbal cue to "try to stand up straighter." Often, by this time, the therapist only needs to walk in front of the client and stand up straight or touch the client's shoulder as a reminder. We typically see changes in sitting and standing posture around Week 3 of the eight-week intervention.

Possible Goals

- Continue to increase strength and range of motion in the hips and the ankles, in order to improve post-stroke balance.

- Improve balance and balance confidence so that clients are beginning to independently use postures at home and engage in more challenging activities at home and in their communities.

- Prepare clients to move to the floor for the next yoga session.

- Continue to connect the breath with movements.

- Remind clients to be in the present moment.

Mantras

Consider a mantra related to a pose, such as when the practice includes Warrior I or II (Virabhadrasana I or II), stating "I am strong, like a warrior," or "Today and every day I am strong, like a warrior." Also, the therapist might consider a mantra about being in the present moment, perhaps something like "I am here now," or "In this moment I am taking care of myself."

Postures and Breath Work

Each posture is completed with the inhale and the exhale; if comfortable, postures may be held for two to three breaths. Postures, breath work, and meditation are presented here in the order that each is to be completed, but this may be modified by the yoga or rehabilitation therapist as necessary.

- Seated:

1. Centering with eyes closed, *state the mantra for today's session.*

2. Take notice of the breath:

    i.   Three-Part Breath (Dirga Pranayama)

    ii. extended exhale

    iii. *repeat the mantra.*

3. Alternate Nostril Breathing (Nadi Shodhana Pranayama).

4. Mudras (wrist, hand, and finger movements with breath).

5. Lateral neck flexion to each side.

6. Neck flexion.

7. Axial Extension (Rekha).

8. Eye exercises, including focusing on a drishti (gazing point).

9. Seated Cat Cow (Chakravakasana).

10. Seated Forward Fold (Upavistha Konasana) (only if not concerned about falling out of the chair).

11. Lion's pose (Simhasana).

12. Seated Spinal Twist (Jathara Parivartanasana) to both sides, arms up towards the ceiling, and axial spinal extension for the transition from one side to the other.

13. Seated Forward Fold (Upavistha Konasana) (only if not concerned about falling out of the chair).

14. Seated Figure 4 or Pigeon (Eka Pada Rajakapotasana), left leg.

15. Ankle/foot movements, left foot.

16. Axial Extension (Rekha).

17. Seated Figure 4 or Pigeon (Eka Pada Rajakapotasana), right leg.

18. Ankle/foot movements, right foot.

19. Seated Forward Fold (Upavistha Konasana) (only if not concerned about falling out of the chair).

- Standing:

    1. Come to standing and move behind the chair to use the back of the chair for support as needed.

    2. Mountain pose (Tadasana).

3. Shoulder rolls, forward and backward.

4. Shoulders to ears.

5. Shoulders down the back.

6. Mountain pose (Tadasana).

7. Cactus arms, arms back down, repeat.

8. Lateral side flexion to each side, one arm up towards the ceiling and the other arm down towards the ground, with axial spinal extension for the transition from one side to the other.

9. Mountain pose (Tadasana).

10. Leg extension (one-legged, modified Locust pose (Salabhasana)), left leg back.

11. Crescent Lunge pose (Anjeneyasana), left leg back.

12. Warrior I (Virabhadrasana I), left leg back.

13. *Repeat the mantra.*

14. Mountain pose (Tadasana).

15. Chair pose (Utkatasana).

16. Mountain pose (Tadasana).

17. Shooting Star (Eka Pada Utthita Tadasana), left leg out.

18. Mountain pose (Tadasana).

19. Five Pointed Star (Utthita Tadasana).

20. Mountain pose (Tadasana).

21. Leg extension (one-legged, modified Locust pose (Salabhasana)), right leg back.

22. Crescent Lunge pose (Anjeneyasana), right leg back.

23. Warrior I (Virabhadrasana I), right leg back.

24. *Repeat the mantra.*

25. Mountain pose (Tadasana).

26. Chair pose (Utkatasana).

27. Mountain pose (Tadasana).

28. Shooting Star (Eka Pada Utthita Tadasana), right leg out.

29. Five Pointed Star (Utthita Tadasana).

30. Mountain pose (Tadasana).

- Seated:

  - Final relaxation and meditation:

  1. Rub the hands together to generate warmth.

  2. Use essential oils if desired.

  3. Place the hands over the eyes and nose.

  4. The hands may stay on the face or in the lap for the relaxation.

  5. *Repeat the mantra.*

  6. Progressive relaxation, going from the toes to the crown of the head, bringing a focus to each body part and then letting it go.

HAND OUT 12.5: GROUP YOGA SESSION IN CHRONIC STROKE: INTERMEDIATE

Follow the sequence from left to right of each row. Start from a seated position.

Seated postures	Center breath work (mantra)	Alternate Nostril Breathing (Nadi Shodhana Pranayama) (mantra)	Mudras
Lateral neck flexion to each side	Neck flexion	Axial Extension (Rekha)	Eye exercises
Cat Cow (Chakravakasana)	Seated Forward Fold (Upavistha Konasana)	Lion's pose (Simhasana)	Spinal Twist (Jathara Parivartanasana), left and right
Seated Forward Fold (Upavistha Konasana)	Figure 4 or Pigeon (Eka Pada Rajakapotasana), left leg	Ankle/foot movements, left foot	Axial Extension (Rekha)
Figure 4 or Pigeon (Eka Pada Rajakapotasana), right leg	Ankle/foot movements, right foot	Seated Forward Fold (Upavistha Konasana)	**Standing postures**

Mountain pose (Tadasana)	Shoulder rolls, forward and back	Shoulders to ears	Shoulders down the back
Mountain pose (Tadasana)	Cactus arms x 2	Lateral flexion, left and right	Mountain pose (Tadasana)
Leg extension, left leg back	Crescent lunge (Anjeneyasana), left leg back	Warrior I (Virabhadrasana I), left leg back (mantra)	Mountain pose (Tadasana)
Chair pose (Utkatasana)	Mountain pose (Tadasana)	Shooting Star (Eka Pada Utthita Tadasana), left leg out	Mountain pose (Tadasana)
Five Pointed Star (Utthita Tadasana)	Mountain pose (Tadasana)	Leg extension, right leg back	Crescent lunge (Anjeneyasana), right leg back
Warrior I (Virabhadrasana I), right leg back (mantra)	Mountain pose (Tadasana)	Chair pose (Utkatasana)	Mountain pose (Tadasana)

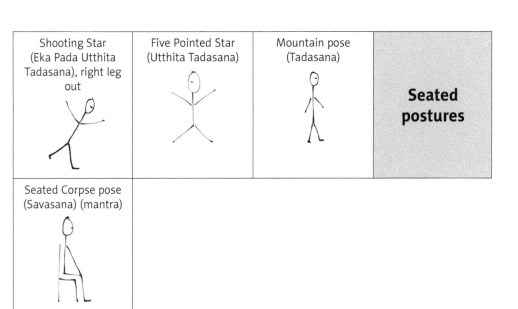

Shooting Star (Eka Pada Utthita Tadasana), right leg out	Five Pointed Star (Utthita Tadasana)	Mountain pose (Tadasana)	**Seated postures**
Seated Corpse pose (Savasana) (mantra)			

ADVANCED PRACTICE WITH SITTING, STANDING, AND FLOOR POSTURES (SESSION 15 OF 16)

Session Notes

- All notes from the One-to-One Yoga Session in a Setting for Clients with Chronic Stroke, the Beginning Group Practice: All in Sitting (Session 2 of 16), and the Intermediate Practice with Standing Postures (Session 8 of 16) are important to review.

- This is the second-to-last practice of the 16 sessions; clients have gained confidence and skills to complete their yoga practice.

- Many of the prior sitting and standing poses have been removed from this practice in order to make time for the transfer to the floor and for the floor postures. This can be altered to best meet the needs of your clients.

- Mountain pose (Tadasana) is commonly used in transitions from one pose to the next during the standing postures. Mountain pose (Tadasana) may be done with the arms down to the side or the arms up in extension over the head, depending on the needs and the abilities of the clients. Having the arms over the head may lead to fatigue or may not be possible with an arm that is hemiparetic.

- Safety in transferring to the floor is paramount and this should only be done if both the therapist and the client feel comfortable and confident in the skills that a floor transfer requires.

  - Use a mat table as necessary and appropriate for clients who are not comfortable with getting to and from the floor.

- Give clients plenty of time and space to complete the transfer; they will not be safe if they feel rushed.

- Use a gait belt for clients who require more assistance to transfer to the floor.

- Remind clients to listen to their bodies, and honor their bodies, in regard to transferring to the floor.

- Remind the staff and the clients that a client may transfer to the floor for one session, but not all sessions, and that this is up to the client and the therapist.

• For clients not moving to the floor, make sure to provide modifications or other poses to be completed in sitting or standing (see Chapter 6).

• Modifications and props may be necessary for postures to be completed on the floor. The therapist must be able to use blocks, bolsters, wedges, or blankets to allow for comfort and decreased risk of injury while moving through the floor postures or resting in Corpse pose (Savasana).

• We only include supine postures in the group chronic stroke practice. We suggest the therapist does not include prone poses on the floor with a group in order to enhance safety and success for all clients.

• Corpse pose (Savasana) is included on the floor for clients who are able to lay on the floor. We like to include eye pillows for clients who wish to have one. Benefits of using an eye pillow during Corpse pose (Savasana) include:

- providing pressure to the eyes, which may relieve tension and eye strain

- blocking light and visual stimuli, allowing for a more restful pose

- possibly helping to calm and rest the mind

- enhancing the integration of the practice into the body

- helping to restore equilibrium.

• As clients with stroke may not be able to physically get their eye pillow and place it correctly on their eyes, we offer the following process to place eye pillows on a client without startling them. First, ask clients who would and would not want assistance with removing glasses and/or placing an eye pillow over the eyes for relaxation in Corpse pose (Savasana). For clients who do wish for assistance, complete the following steps.

- As clients are preparing for Corpse pose (Savasana), remind them that the therapist or assistants will come round to place an eye pillow on each individual.

- If a client prefers to not receive an eye pillow, they can tell the therapist or raise their hand.

- Quietly approach the client once they are on the floor and situated for Corpse pose (Savasana); quietly tell them that you are there and will place the mask on their eyes.

- If they would like assistance, remove their glasses as necessary and let the client know where the glasses have been placed (in the shirt pocket, on their chest; *not* on the floor, where they could be rolled on).

- Unless requested otherwise, gently place the eye pillow over the eyes, pressing lightly on the eyes and sliding the fingers away from the nose.

Possible Goals

- Continue to increase standing and sitting posture.

- Improve confidence and the ability to transfer to and from the floor.

- Engage in supine postures, including Corpse pose (Savasana).

- Improve lower extremity strength, range of motion, and balance.

- Continue to be in the present moment and connect the breath with movement.

- Embed yoga practices and breath work into daily activities or during stressful situations.

Mantras

Clients in the advanced group practice have likely demonstrated improvements or changes in their post-stroke impairments. They may be thankful or excited for their progress, and the therapist may wish to include mantras such as "I am grateful for all that my mind and my body can do," or "Every day we can do more and we are whole."

Postures and Breath Work

Each posture is completed with the inhale and the exhale; if comfortable, postures may be held for two to three breaths. Postures, breath work, and meditation are presented here in the order that each is to be completed, but this may be modified by the yoga or rehabilitation therapist as necessary.

- Seated:

    1. Centering with eyes closed, *state the mantra for today's session.*

    2. Take notice of the breath.

    i.   Three-Part Breath (Dirga Pranayama)

    ii.   extended exhale

    iii.   *repeat the mantra.*

3. Alternate Nostril Breathing (Nadi Shodhana Pranayama).

4. Mudras (wrist, hand, and finger movements with breath).

5. Lateral neck flexion to each side.

6. Neck flexion.

7. Axial Extension (Rekha).

8. Eye exercises.

9. Seated Cat Cow (Chakravakasana).

10. Seated Forward Fold (Upavistha Konasana) (only if not concerned about falling out of the chair).

- Standing:

  1. Come to standing and move behind the chair.

  2. For support in standing use:

     − the back of the chair for support as needed

     − the wall

     − nothing, if this is appropriate and safe.

  3. Mountain pose (Tadasana).

  4. Shoulder rolls, forward and backward.

  5. Mountain pose (Tadasana).

  6. Lateral side flexion to each side, one arm up towards the ceiling and the other arm down towards the ground, with axial spinal extension for the transition from one side to the other.

  7. Mountain pose (Tadasana).

  8. Lion's pose (Simhasana) while standing and holding on to the chair.

  9. Mountain pose (Tadasana).

  10. Leg extension (one-legged, modified Locust pose (Salabhasana)), left leg back.

  11. Warrior I (Virabhadrasana I), left leg back.

12. Mountain pose (Tadasana).

13. Leg extension (one-legged, modified Locust pose (Salabhasana)), right leg back.

14. Warrior I (Virabhadrasana I), right leg back.

15. Mountain pose (Tadasana).

16. Shooting Star (Eka Pada Utthita Tadasana), left leg out.

17. Mountain pose (Tadasana).

18. Shooting Star (Eka Pada Utthita Tadasana), right leg out.

19. Mountain pose (Tadasana).

20. Chair pose (Utkatasana).

21. *Repeat the mantra.*

22. Mountain pose (Tadasana).

23. Tree pose (Vrksasana), including focusing on a drishti (gazing point), left leg grounded and right foot up.

24. Mountain pose (Tadasana).

25. Tree pose (Vrksasana), including focusing on a drishti (gazing point), right leg grounded and left foot up.

Transfer to the floor for floor postures in supine:

- Supine poses:

  1. Knees to Chest (Apanasana), head turns to left and right.

  2. Bridge pose (Setu Bandha Sarvangasana).

  3. Anterior and Posterior Hip Tilts.

  4. Supine on floor with knees bent, resting pose.

  5. Figure 4 or Pigeon (Eka Pada Rajakapotasana), left leg.

  6. Ankle/foot movements, left leg.

  7. Supine on floor with knees bent, resting pose.

  8. Figure 4 or Pigeon (Eka Pada Rajakapotasana), right leg.

  9. Ankle/foot movements, right leg.

  10. Supine on floor with knees bent, resting pose.

11. Spinal Twists (Jathara Parivartanasana) with knees bent, to both the left and the right.

12. Knees to Chest (Apanasana) or simply hug the knees.

13. Big Toe pose (Padangusthasana), using yoga strap or gait belt, left leg to the ceiling, left leg into abduction.

14. Transition yoga strap or gait belt to other leg.

15. Supine on floor with knees bent, resting pose if needed.

16. Big Toe pose (Padangusthasana), using yoga strap or gait belt, right leg to the ceiling, right leg into abduction.

- Final relaxation and meditation:

  1. Corpse pose (Savasana) with eye pillow.

  2. Three-Part Breath (Dirga Pranayama).

  3. *Repeat the mantra.*

  4. Progressive relaxation, going from the toes to the crown of the head, bringing a focus to each body part and then letting it go.

HAND OUT 12.6: GROUP YOGA SESSION IN CHRONIC STROKE: ADVANCED

Follow the sequence from left to right of each row. Start from a seated position.

	Center breath work (mantra)	Alternate Nostril Breathing (Nadi Shodhana Pranayama) (mantra)	Mudras
Seated postures			
Lateral neck flexion to each side	Neck flexion	Axial Extension (Rekha)	Eye exercise
Cat Cow (Chakravakasana)	Seated Forward Fold (Upavistha Konasana)	**Standing postures**	Mountain pose (Tadasana)
Shoulder rolls, forward and backward	Mountain pose (Tadasana)	Lateral side flexion to each side	Mountain pose (Tadasana)
Lion's pose (Simhasana)	Mountain pose (Tadasana)	Leg extension, left leg back	Warrior I (Virabhadrasana I), left leg back

Mountain pose (Tadasana)	Warrior I (Virabhadrasana I), right leg back	Mountain pose (Tadasana)	Shooting Star (Eka Pada Utthita Tadasana), left leg out
Mountain pose (Tadasana)	Chair pose (Utkatasana) (mantra)	Mountain pose (Tadasana)	Tree pose (Vrksasana), right foot up
Mountain pose (Tadasana)	Tree pose (Vrksasana), left foot up	**Supine floor postures**	Knees to Chest (Apanasana)
Bridge pose (Setu Bandha Sarvangasana)	Hip tilts	Supine on floor, knees bent, resting pose	Figure 4 or Pigeon (Eka Pada Rajakapotasana), left leg
Ankle/foot movements, left foot	Supine on floor, knees bent, resting pose	Figure 4 or Pigeon (Eka Pada Rajakapotasana), right leg	Ankle/foot movements, right foot

Supine on floor, knees bent, resting pose	Spinal Twist (Jathara Parivartanasana), both sides	Knees to Chest (Apanasana)	Big Toe pose (Padangusthasana), abduction, left leg
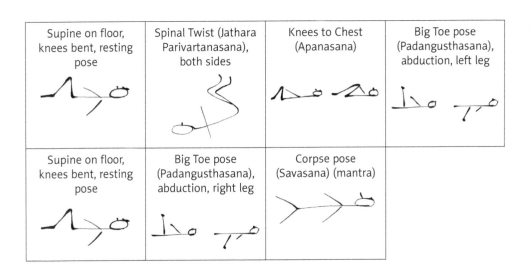			
Supine on floor, knees bent, resting pose	Big Toe pose (Padangusthasana), abduction, right leg	Corpse pose (Savasana) (mantra)	

SAMPLE RESTORATIVE PRACTICE 1

Session Notes

- Props required for this practice per person: two blocks, two to four blankets, two bolsters, one eye pillow, one strap, one sandbag.

- Poses last 5–20 minutes and can be modified based on need, comfort, or other time requirements.

- Restorative practices generally improve clarity in the mind, improve breathing and circulation, and provide a deeper level of relaxation than sleep!

- This sequence is a primarily reclining sequence. Poses can be mixed and matched with other restorative sequences. However, it is important to avoid postures where the head is lower than the heart. These are considered inversions, and an inverted posture causes the heart to work harder and the blood pressure to rise. This is not an issue in individuals with healthy cardiovascular systems, but in individuals with a recent insult to the cardiovascular system, this could create a problem. As a result, avoid all inverted poses that are held for any period of time (which is all restorative poses since they are typically held for up to 20 minutes).

- Restorative practices should be conducted in a quiet environment, as the purpose of a restorative practice is relaxation. Avoid conducting a restorative practice in a noisy or busy environment. A patient room or chapel may be an ideal place for the restorative practice to take place.

- Restorative poses stimulate the relaxation response and enhance healing in the body. While patients may not feel they are "working" in restorative yoga, or believe in the motto "no pain, no gain," it is important to express to them the need their body has for repair, which is facilitated during restorative yoga.

- These restorative poses can be conducted on the floor, on a mat table, and, as a last resort, in the patient's bed.

- Use a gait belt to transfer the patient as needed from sitting to standing or to transfer to the floor.

Possible Goals

- Understand the need for relaxation in stroke recovery.

- Integrate yoga into daily recovery, even rest days.

- Describe the benefits of restorative yoga.

Mantras

In restorative yoga, clients may have trouble coming to stillness or accepting that resting can be beneficial. Mantras that may be fitting in this scenario include "My body is grateful for rest," or "Rest helps my body and brain heal."

Postures and Breath Work

1. Alternate Nostril Breathing (Nadi Shodhana Pranayama) (3 minutes).

2. Basic Relaxation Asana (10 minutes).

3. Queen's pose (Salamba Baddha Konasana) (15 minutes).

4. Side Resting pose with bolster (10 minutes—5 minutes on each side).

5. Supported Reclining Bound Angle pose (Supta Baddha Konasana) (15 minutes).

6. Corpse pose (Savasana) (7 minutes).

HAND OUT 12.7: RESTORATIVE PRACTICE 1

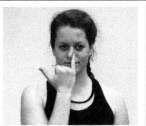

Alternate Nostril Breathing (Nadi Shodhana Pranayama) (3 minutes)	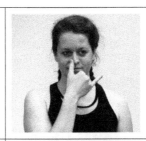
Basic Relaxation pose (10 minutes)	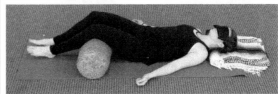
Queen's pose (Salamba Baddha Konasana) (15 minutes)	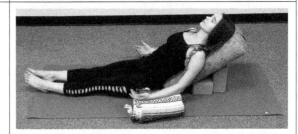
Side Lying "Spooning" pose (10 minutes—5 minutes on each side)	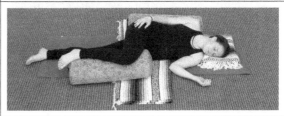
Supported Bound Angle pose (15 minutes)	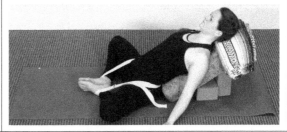
Corpse pose (Savasana) (7 minutes)	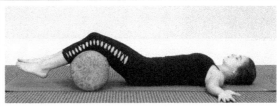

SAMPLE RESTORATIVE PRACTICE 2

Session Notes

- This sequence is a primarily seated or forward folding sequence. Poses can be mixed and matched with other restorative sequences. However, it is important to avoid postures where the head is lower than the heart. These are considered inversions, and an inverted posture causes the heart to work harder and the blood pressure to rise. This is not an issue in individuals with healthy cardiovascular systems, but in individuals with a recent insult to the cardiovascular system, this could create a problem. As a result, avoid all inverted poses that are held for any period of time (which is all restorative poses since they are typically held for up to 20 minutes).

- Props required for this practice per person: two blankets, two bolsters, one eye pillow, one sandbag.

- Poses last 5–20 minutes and can be modified based on need, comfort, or other time requirements.

- Restorative practices generally improve clarity in the mind, improve breathing and circulation, and provide a deeper level of relaxation than sleep!

- Restorative practices should be conducted in a quiet environment, as the purpose of a restorative practice is relaxation. Avoid conducting a restorative practice in a noisy or busy environment. A patient room or chapel may be an ideal place for the restorative practice to take place.

- Restorative poses stimulate the relaxation response and enhance healing in the body. While patients may not feel they are "working" in restorative yoga, or believe in the motto "no pain, no gain," it is important to express to them the need their body has for repair, which is facilitated during restorative yoga.

- These restorative poses can be conducted on the floor, on a mat table, and, as a last resort, in the patient's bed.

- Use a gait belt to transfer the patient as needed from sitting to standing or to transfer to the floor.

Possible Goals

- The client will understand the need for relaxation in stroke recovery.

- The client will learn to integrate yoga into daily recovery.

- The client will be able to describe the benefits of restorative yoga.

Mantras

In restorative yoga, clients may have trouble coming to stillness or accepting that resting can be beneficial. Mantras that may be fitting in this scenario include "My body is grateful for rest," or "Rest helps my body and brain heal."

Postures and Breath Work

1. Upright Seated Cat (Marjariasana) and Cow (Bitilasana)—Cat Cow (Chakravakasana) (5 rotations over 2 minutes).

2. Supported Wide-Angle Seated Forward Fold (Upavistha Konasana) (10 minutes).

3. Reclining Twist with a Bolster (10 minutes—5 minutes on each side).

4. Restorative Child's pose (Restorative Balasana) on bolsters (10 minutes).

5. Seated Angle pose (5 minutes).

6. Add Bee Breath (Bhramari Pranayama) (5 minutes) to Seated Angle pose.

7. Corpse pose (Savasana) (8 minutes).

HAND OUT 12.8: RESTORATIVE PRACTICE 2

Upright Seated Cat (Marjariasana) and Cow (Bitilasana)—Cat Cow (Chakravakasana) (5 rotations over 2 minutes)	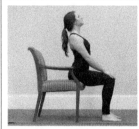 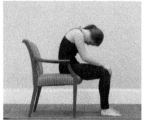
Supported Wide-Angle Seated Forward Fold (Upavistha Konasana) (10 minutes)	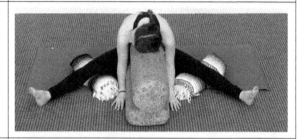
Reclining Twist with a Bolster (10 minutes—5 minutes on each side)	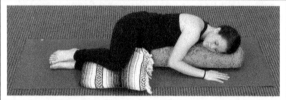
Restorative Child's pose (Restorative Balasana) on bolsters (10 minutes)	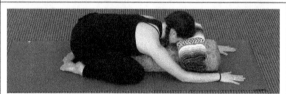
Seated Angle pose (5 minutes) Bee Breath (Bhramari Pranayama) (5 minutes) in Seated Angle pose	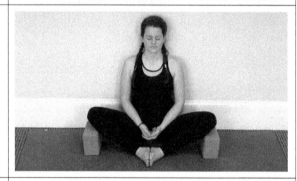
Corpse pose (Savasana) (8 minutes)	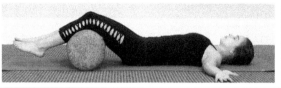

CHAPTER 13

Tips and Resources to Best Integrate Yoga into Practice

It can be challenging to truly integrate yoga into practice or the community or to develop the best yoga session for clients with stroke. In this chapter we pull together resources that we hope are helpful to yoga teachers, yoga therapists, and rehabilitation therapists who are using yoga with clients with stroke. We include forms and hand outs that can be replicated or found at our website: www.mergingyogaandrehabilitation. com. In this chapter we include:

- stroke resources, including excellent websites about post-stroke disability

- information about the dose of yoga

- an attendance form to track client attendance in yoga sessions

- a form to track whether the yoga or rehabilitation therapist is delivering the yoga intervention as planned (fidelity checklist)

- tips for enhancing communication after a stroke

- top-ten tips for delivering yoga as a part of clinical practice

- a hand out that includes the perceived benefits of yoga postures, breath work, meditations, and mudras

- "tips of the trade," including information about documentation and billing

- tips to develop community-based yoga sites for people with disabilities

- basic information about yoga for the caregiver who is helping the client after their stroke

- book and internet resources about yoga and yoga therapy.

Stroke Resources

There are many resources that the therapist can access to help provide information about a stroke. When working with clients with stroke and their family and friends, it is important to provide evidence that supports the information or training being provided or encouraged. Information regarding stroke, the effects of stroke, rehabilitation, and many other aspects of stroke recovery may be found at the following websites:

- www.stroke.org.uk
- www.strokeassociation.org/STROKEORG
- www.stroke.org
- www.world-stroke.org
- https://strokefoundation.org.au.

For more information about the changes or the effects of stroke that may occur, see information online at www.stroke.org.uk/what-stroke/common-problems-after-stroke or www.worldstrokecampaign.org/learn/disorders-after-stroke.html. Understanding the impact of stroke will help the yoga or rehabilitation therapist to deliver yoga in a more safe and effective way and allow the therapist to tailor it to the needs of the individual with stroke.

Is More Yoga Better? Let's Consider Dosing of Yoga

Dosing of yoga has rarely been studied, and dosing of rehabilitation (occupational therapy, physical therapy, recreational therapy, speech therapy) after stroke is often not addressed in studies. The dose of an intervention, whether it is yoga or some other aspect of rehabilitation, typically includes things like the frequency, duration, and intensity of the intervention (Page, Schmid, and Harris 2012). In our studies for people with chronic stroke we have included 16 sessions of yoga. The yoga was delivered in one-hour increments twice a week for eight weeks; therefore participants were offered approximately 16 hours of yoga over the eight weeks. We often begin to see a change in posture and other aspects of physical recovery in around Week 3. While there have not been enough studies to prove the correct dose of yoga after a stroke, we do see that people who have better attendance also seem to have better outcomes, seemingly regardless of diagnosis. After stroke, the improved outcomes with increased attendance are seen throughout the cognitive, emotional, and physical abilities; however, we tend to see physical improvements first. In our research studies, it appears that it may take longer, or increased attendance at yoga sessions, to see improvements in cognitive or emotional changes, such as improved confidence or processing of information. With time, we even see changes in aphasia, with study participants showing improved processing of information and ability to speak more words! We also see changes in reading, in both the ability to read and comprehension of the information, after 16 sessions of yoga. In our most recent study (not yet published), we provided up to 24 weeks of yoga to people with chronic pain (some of the participants also had a stroke) who were patients at a pain clinic. The medical doctors and administration were so happy with the results, including decreased pain-related disability, that they continued to offer yoga, for free, to the study participants. We recently completed interviews with approximately ten of the original study participants who have now received over two years of yoga. Those individuals talked about how they really noticed many physical changes in their bodies in the first two to six months of yoga. Importantly though, they felt that cognitive and emotional changes did not happen until about nine months to a year into the yoga intervention. Therefore, while not proven, we do believe that more is better when it comes to yoga. This amount or dose of yoga cannot, of course, be delivered in a typical rehabilitation setting, but it is possible in the community, when supported by adaptive yoga, and offers an inexpensive yoga.

We recommend that yoga and rehabilitation therapists track attendance in regard to yoga and what is accomplished during the yoga intervention. Hand Out 13.1 can be used to track attendance. This form was developed for a 16-session yoga intervention, but can be modified as needed.

HAND OUT 13.1: ATTENDANCE FORM TO TRACK YOGA SESSIONS

Name:				
Session	**Date**	**Attend?**	**Fully participate?**	**Follow up, reason for not attending**
1		Yes / No	Yes / No / Medium	
2		Yes / No	Yes / No / Medium	
3		Yes / No	Yes / No / Medium	
4		Yes / No	Yes / No / Medium	
5		Yes / No	Yes / No / Medium	
6		Yes / No	Yes / No / Medium	
7		Yes / No	Yes / No / Medium	
8		Yes / No	Yes / No / Medium	
9		Yes / No	Yes / No / Medium	
10		Yes / No	Yes / No / Medium	
11		Yes / No	Yes / No / Medium	
12		Yes / No	Yes / No / Medium	
13		Yes / No	Yes / No / Medium	
14		Yes / No	Yes / No / Medium	
15		Yes / No	Yes / No / Medium	
16		Yes / No	Yes / No / Medium	

Is the Yoga or Rehabilitation Therapist Delivering the Planned Intervention?

In both research and clinical practice, we plan to deliver a certain intervention with specific components. It is helpful to assess the fidelity of the delivery of the intervention. Measuring fidelity allows us to know the extent to which the intervention was delivered in a way that adheres to the planned or established protocol. We have assessed fidelity in a number of our yoga studies and provided a form in Hand Out 13.2 for therapists to assess the fidelity of their delivery of the yoga intervention. This is only an example, and the therapist may want to assess the delivery of different components of the yoga intervention that is planned for the client. This may be as simple or complicated as the yoga or rehabilitation therapist wishes to make it.

HAND OUT 13.2: FIDELITY CHECKLIST FORM

Aspect of intervention	Completed?	Other comments or things to remember?
Physical postures	☐ Yes ☐ No ☐ Some	
Connected breath to movement	☐ Yes ☐ No ☐ Some	
Relaxation/meditation	☐ Yes ☐ No ☐ Some	
Affirmations	☐ Yes ☐ No ☐ Some	
Planned physical components (i.e. chair, standing, floor)	☐ Yes ☐ No ☐ Some	
Vitals assessed (may include blood pressure or heart rate as necessary or appropriate)	☐ Yes ☐ No ☐ Some	
Other	☐ Yes ☐ No ☐ Some	

Tips for Enhancing Communication After a Stroke

As discussed in Chapter 2, there are many things that happen after a stroke, and communication is commonly impacted. When working with someone with aphasia or other communication issues, consider using the following tips to enhance communication during yoga and therapy.

- Respect the client with aphasia.

- Remember that aphasia is not necessarily associated with changes in intelligence.

- Remain patient with each other.

- Watch the volume of the voice—it is natural to increase one's volume when a client does not understand, but it is important to understand they do not (necessarily) have a hearing impairment just because their comprehension is impaired.

- Give simple, one- or two-step instructions; work on one idea at a time.

- Use simple, clear speech.

- Speak slowly and articulate each word.

- Allow ample time for the client with stroke to process the information and to follow the instruction or respond.

- Remember that the client with stroke may understand what the therapist is saying and follow the directions but not be able to verbally respond with the correct words.

- Make conversations easier by using drawings or writing things down.

- Consider using photos or maps if it would help communication.

- Use pointing or other cues.

- Use simple, tactile cues as appropriate (i.e. touch the left arm if the instruction is to raise the left arm).

- Make sure the client understands the words or directions from the therapist and understands what the therapist is asking or directing them to do.

- Remind caregivers to follow these tips as well. This may enhance communication during the hospital stay or at home after discharge from the hospital.

- Check out this website for additional ideas and tips for communicating with clients who have sustained a stroke: www.stroke.org/we-can-help/survivors/stroke-recovery/post-stroke-conditions/physical/aphasia.

Top-Ten Tips for Delivering Yoga as a Part of Rehabilitation After a Stroke

We have learned a lot of things from a lot of people in regard to how to safely and effectively include yoga after stroke. In the following list, we include the top-ten things that we have learned from talking to yoga and rehabilitation therapists and from our previous research studies.

1. **Have a personal yoga practice** that includes daily or at least weekly practices. This is a common part of yoga teacher trainings—that yoga teachers should include daily or weekly yoga practices. Yogic philosophies indicate that one cannot deliver yoga in a safe and effective manner if the teacher has not embedded yoga into her or his own life.

2. **Complete additional training** and either become a yoga teacher or take continuing education courses specific to stroke or yoga as an intervention in rehabilitation. The therapist must know what they are doing and why something is being done with an individual client.

3. Throughout the stroke recovery trajectory, it is important to **include physical poses that address the asymmetry** that may occur in the body after a stroke. When appropriate, do not be afraid to **move people into quadruped** (all fours). Consider Table Top (Goasana), Balancing Table Top (contralateral movements of the arms and legs in Table Top), Cat Cow (Chakravakasana), or Child's pose (Balasana).

4. **Use extension poses**, such as Warrior I (Virabhadrasana I) or Crescent Lunge (Anjeneyasana), to increase energy. People with stroke often suffer from fatigue throughout their recovery and many years into the future. Increasing energy through yoga may be very helpful to many clients with stroke.

5. In seated and standing postures, it will often be necessary for the yoga or rehabilitation therapist to **encourage Axial Extension (Rekha)**—sitting up straight, with the crown or the top of the head towards the ceiling. To do this, the therapist or yoga teacher may place the right hand on the middle of the back and lightly press forward, and, at the same time, place the left hand on the left shoulder and lightly pull back. Use verbal and tactile cueing to see improvements. The encouragement of active Axial Extension (Rekha) is necessary after stroke. We commonly see people slouched over and they need verbal and tactile cueing to sit up straighter. This slouched position is likely related to an increased amount of sedentary time sitting in a wheelchair or other chair. The sedentary time in a supported seated position leads to muscle weakness and muscle memory of the slouched position. We have seen dramatic changes with enhanced Axial Extension (Rekha) in as little as three weeks of yoga with clients after a stroke. See Figure 13.1 for photos of the therapist using tactile cueing to enhance Axial Extension (Rekha).

6. **Include hip openers in sitting, standing, and floor yoga postures.** Due to the increased time in seated postures that is common after stroke, the hip flexors become very tight or shortened. Include modified lunges or Warrior I or Warrior II (Virabhadrasana I or Virabhadrasana II). Warrior II (Virabhadrasana II) helps to open the hip flexors and strengthen the muscles in the leg. Participants in our stroke and yoga research studies have reported that they think that the modified Warrior I (Virabhadrasana I) pose was the most helpful to them in terms of improving their walking ability and endurance.

7. **Include mantras during practice**, such as "I am strong enough," "I am whole enough," "I am enough," or "I am able." Clients with stroke often do not feel whole or lament the person they "used to be." We have found mantras to be helpful in the healing and recovery process. When facing new challenges, individuals in our studies often report the daily use of a mantra learned in yoga to remind themselves of their strength and abilities.

8. **Tailor the practice to meet the individual needs of the client.** Not all individuals with stroke are the same or have the same post-stroke needs. It is best to meet their needs by talking with them and their family and tailoring their yoga practice or yoga therapy to best address their abilities, their needs, and their goals. While we included yoga practices with specific postures in this book, the therapist must assess the needs and abilities of the client to best serve them in their yoga practice or therapy.

9. **Use props and modifications as necessary** so that the person with stroke always feels successful in their practice. This takes skill and practice, both in the verbal and tactile cueing and in the correct and safe use of props. Props may include traditional yoga props, such as straps, blocks, or bolsters, but may also include more traditional rehabilitation props, such as gait or transfer belts, elevated mat tables, wedges, or a leg lifter.

10. **It is all right if the client with stroke does fall asleep during Corpse pose (Savasana).** Corpse pose (Savasana) is the time to allow the body to integrate the yoga practice. While it is best for the client to stay awake during Corpse pose (Savasana) and focus on the meditation or the breath, we know it is common for people to be fatigued after the yoga practice and fall asleep.

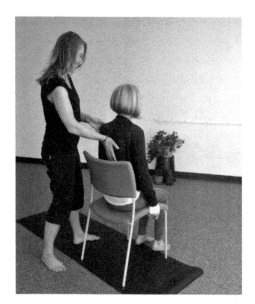 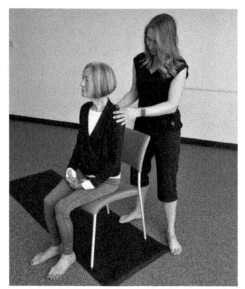

Figure 13.1

Benefits of Yoga

It is important for the therapist to know and understand why to choose a certain asana or pranayama for each client. Hand Out 13.3 is a quick reference guide that includes the name of the posture or breath work in both English and Sanskrit and the perceived benefits of each practice. The list is in alphabetical order by English names.

HAND OUT 13.3: QUICK REFERENCE GUIDE TO POSES, BREATH WORK, AND THE BENEFITS OF EACH

Selected pranayama and yoga poses	Sanskrit name	Perceived benefits
Pranayama or breathing practices		
Alternate Nostril Breathing	Nadi Shodhana Pranayama	• Stimulates and harmonizes both sides of the hemispheres of the brain, which is important after damage to the brain • Activates the parasympathetic nervous system • Decreases blood pressure • Improves attention and fine motor coordination
Bee Breath	Bhramari Pranayama	• Calms the mind • Helps to reduce blood pressure • Improves feelings of fatigue
Bellows Breath	Bhastrika Pranayama	• Improves circulation (and oxygenates blood) through the entire body • Energizes the body
Breath of Fire/ Skull Shining Breath	Kapalabhati Pranayama	• Energizing and invigorating • Improves circulation (and oxygenates blood) through the entire body • Detoxifies and cleanses the body, improves digestion
Coordinate breath with movements Three-Part Breath Slower and extended exhales, pushing the breath out at the bottom of exhale	Dirga Pranayama	• Decreases blood pressure • Increases oxygenation throughout the body and strengthens respiratory system • Detoxifies and cleanses the body • Triggers the "relaxation response," interrupts stress reaction, tips the nervous system into the peripheral nervous system, allows for rest, renewal, and healing • Strengthens low belly muscles
NA	Viloma Pranayama	• Helps to reduce anxiety and tension • Can be used to cool the body • May enhance control of breath
Asana or yoga postures		
Big Toe pose, supine on floor, posterior leg stretches, to the ceiling and to the side (abduction)	Padangusthasana	• Known to relieve back pain • Stretches hamstrings, hip adductors, and calf muscles • Strengthens knees • Supports proper pelvic position—levelness • May decrease blood pressure

Selected pranayama and yoga poses	Sanskrit name	Perceived benefits
Boat pose	Navasana	• Improves balance • Improves digestion • Decreases stress • Improves confidence
Bridge pose	Setu Bandha Sarvangasana	• Stretches muscles and connective tissue in the front of the body • Strengthens the muscles in the posterior body • Improves alignment in the hips/knees/ankles/feet • Strengthens the arches of the feet, improving balance • Calming and reduces stress • Improves digestion
Cat Cow	Cat: Marjariasana Cow: Bitilasana Cat Cow: Chakravakasana	• Awakens the spine • Energizes, due to the back extension • Improves sitting and standing posture • Enhances coordination • Stretches and strengthens the front and back of the body
Chair pose	Utkatasana	• Enhances balance • Strengthens the leg muscles • Stretches the muscles of the chest and shoulders • Stimulates the heart and diaphragm
Child's pose	Balasana	• Passive stretch to the back of the body and a stretch to the hips, thighs, and ankles • Reduces stress • Reduces fatigue
Cobra pose	Bhujangasana	• Strengthens and stretches the arm, shoulder, and upper back muscles • Improves lower back flexibility and stiffness • Energizes, due to the back bend • Improves the mood
Corpse pose or "Constructive Rest Pose" (knees bent and bound together, feet flat on floor)	Savasana	• Most safe and relaxed position for Corpse pose (Savasana) (versus sitting in a chair) • Can utilize an eye pillow • Lumbar spine opens with the knees bent • Ideal position for deep, guided relaxation • Relaxes the body • Allows time for the mind and the body to integrate the practice • Lowers blood pressure

Crescent Lunge pose	Anjeneyasana	• Stretches the hip flexors (psoas), which are very tight secondary to the amount of sitting that is common after stroke, which may be related to improved gait and endurance • Increases hip extension, calf flexibility, and ankle dorsiflexion: all known to reduce falls • Opens the hips • Stretches the muscles and connective tissue of the anterior body, which shorten with prolonged sitting • Strengthens the muscles in the posterior/back of the body, which get weak and overstretched from prolonged sitting • Increases confidence and self-esteem
Downward Facing Dog	Adho Mukha Svanasana	• Calming and energizing • Proprioceptive feedback to all limbs • Strengthens and stretches the muscles in the front and the back of the body • Improves confidence • May be done at the wall for acute stroke or if the client is not ready for the full posture
Easy pose	Sukhasana	• Hip opener • Improves posture • Strengthens the back muscles • Stretches the muscles of the hips, knees, and ankles • Decreases stress and anxiety
Extended Side Angle pose	Utthita Parsvakonasana	• Deep stretch to the groin muscles and the hamstrings • Improves balance • Strengthens the lower extremity muscles • Stretches the intercostal muscles and the abdominal muscles • Increases stamina and energy
Eye activity, holding the eyes steady on a particular point, the drishti (focal point)	NA	• Steady eyes = steady mind; the mind and the thoughts may be stilled as the eyes hold steady • Increases balance, reduces falls
Eye movements to the left and the right, up and down, and in figure 8	NA	• Crosses the midline • Promotes the repair of brain tissue and development of alternate pathways (think neuroplasticity) • Enhances communication between the two hemispheres of the brain • Improves coordination

Selected pranayama and yoga poses	Sanskrit name	Perceived benefits
Figure 4 or Pigeon with ankle/foot/toes range of motion, in sitting or supine	Eka Pada Rajakapotasana	• Strengthens and stretches all the leg, thigh, and hip muscles • Reduces falls and improves balance by increasing strength, flexibility, and coordination • "Educates" and awakens feet, potentially improving sensory impairment • Stretches the hip and glute muscles, including the piriformis muscle • Releases pressure in the low back
Five Pointed Star pose or Shooting Star pose	Utthita Tadasana or Eka Pada Utthita Tadasana	• Improves balance • Improves strength in the lower extremities • Five Pointed Star (Utthita Tadasana) is grounding and energizing • Shooting Star (Eka Pada Utthita Tadasana) is energizing
Forward Fold (while seated in chair or on floor)	Upavistha Konasana	• Soothes the lumbar spine by stretching, lengthening, and increasing circulation • Stretches and relaxes the hips and buttocks • Strengthens the thighs • Massages the digestive organs • Strengthens breathing by providing pressure/obstruction • Pressure on the diaphragm, which may decrease blood pressure
Goddess pose (or Fierce Angle pose)	Utkata Konasana	• Strengthens and stretches the muscles of the lower extremities • Stimulates and strengthens the muscles of the pelvic floor • Hip opener
Hand to opposite knee, slight rotation/twist	NA	• Strengthens the thigh muscles • Crosses the midline • Improves coordination • Stimulates brain hemispheric communication through bilateral stimulation and crossing the midline • Neutralizer for previous challenging work of the hips, knees, and feet before coming to standing
Happy Baby or Dead Bug pose	Ananda Balasana	• Hip opener • Stretches the groin and inner thigh muscles • Releases the low back and decreases back pain • Quiets the mind • Decreases stress

Head, neck movements; flexion, Axial Extension (Rekha), later flexion	Axial Extension: Rekha	• Relaxes head, shoulder, and neck tension • Increases circulation • Opens the sinuses and inner ears • Reduces the risk of respiratory and ear infections • Stimulates brain tissue by increasing cerebral spinal fluid movement • Enhances communication between the two hemispheres of the brain • Centers and hydrates the cervical disks • Counteracts effects of slumping, reduces headaches and other problems caused by a "head forward" position
Knees to Chest pose	Apanasana	• Stabilizes while stretching the muscles of the pelvis and the low back • Reduces low back pain • Decreases blood pressure • Decreases anxiety
Lion's pose	Simhasana	• Relieves tension and stress • Stretches and strengthens the face muscles, which are often impacted after stroke and linked to dysarthria • Energizing and awaking • Eases the mind
Locust pose, modified in standing, hip extensions, pelvis remains unmoved or on the floor in prone	Salabhasana	• Increases posterior muscle strength • Stretches the hip flexors, which are likely to shorten with prolonged sitting after stroke • Increases inferior bone density • Improves balance, grace, and confidence
Mountain pose	Tadasana	• Improves posture and balance • Strengthens lower extremity muscles • Steadies breathing and increases awareness
Plank	Kumbhakasana	• Strengthens the muscles around the spine • Strengthens the arm, chest, and back muscles
Scapular, shoulder range of motion and arm movements	NA	• Releases shoulder and neck tension • Increases circulation to the entire upper body, reduces upper back pain and tightness • Counteracts the effects of slumping • Reduces headaches caused by shoulder tension • Stretches, strengthens, and relaxes arms, wrists, hands, shoulders, back, and chest

Selected pranayama and yoga poses	Sanskrit name	Perceived benefits
Sphinx pose	Salamba Bhujangasana	• Strengthens and stretches the muscles of the front of the body • Strengthens the spinal muscles • Energizes, due to the back bend • Improves the mood • Improves fatigue
Spinal movements: extension, flexion, lateral flexion	NA	• Releases strain and tension • Increases strength and flexibility in the back muscles, stretches the lower back • Centers and hydrates the intervertebral disks • Increases cerebrospinal fluid movement/circulation • Stimulates and tones the nervous system • Soothes and nourishes the "stress responders," our adrenal glands and the entire endocrine system • Helps encourage the release of bottled-up emotions • Improves circulation to the abdominal organs, cleansing, stimulating, toning and massaging, improving digestion and elimination and general functioning • Tones the pelvic muscles for a centered, level, supportive pelvis
Spinal Twist	Jathara Parivartanasana	• Releases pressure in the low back • Improves digestion • Quiets the mind
Standing Forward Fold	Uttanasana	• Improves balance • Stretches the muscles in the back of the body • Strengthens the thighs and the knees
Table Top or quadruped	Goasana	• Strengthens and aligns the spine • Is considered therapeutic and is commonly used in therapy • Helps with asymmetry, which is common after stroke • Gives proprioceptive feedback into the limb that has hemiparesis • Is grounding to the client

Toe/ball of foot lifts with small knee bends with the feet flat on the floor	NA	• "Awakens" the lower extremities, potentially bringing awareness to the feet and ankles • Places some "demand" on the muscles to strengthen them • Improves leg/foot/ankle alignment • Increases bone density • Improves balance
Transferring to and from the floor	NA	• Improves the ability to get up and down from the floor safely • Increases confidence in the ability to get up if/when there is a fall • Improves confidence to go to the floor by choice, for activities such as yoga, playing with children, gardening
Tree pose	Vrksasana	• Improves and challenges balance • Stretches and strengthens the lower extremity muscles • Strengthens the ankles
Upward Facing Dog	Urdha Mukha Svanasana	• Improves postures • Strengthens and stretches the muscles of the front of the body • Strengthens the spinal muscles • Opens the chest, sternum, and muscles that surround the rib cage • Energizes, due to the back bend • Improves the mood • Improves fatigue
Warrior I	Virabhadrasana I	• Stretches the hip flexors (psoas), which are very tight secondary to the amount of sitting that is common after stroke; may be related to improved gait and endurance; increases hip extension, calf flexibility, and ankle dorsiflexion: all known to reduce falls • Opens the hips • Stretches the muscles and connective tissue of the anterior body, which shorten with prolonged sitting • Strengthens the muscles in the posterior/back of the body, which get weak and overstretched from prolonged sitting • Increases confidence and self-esteem • Improves focus and balance • Improves circulation • When the arms are up (and not using the chair for balance), there is potential for strengthening and stretching the shoulders and arms • Energizes, due to the back extension

Selected pranayama and yoga poses	Sanskrit name	Perceived benefits
Warrior II	Virabhadrasana II	• Stretches the hip flexors (psoas), which are very tight secondary to the amount of sitting that is common after stroke; may be related to improved gait and endurance; increases hip extension, calf flexibility, and ankle dorsiflexion: all known to reduce falls • Improves balance and strength • Improves circulation and is energizing • Grounding
Warrior III	Virabhadrasana III	• Strengthens the back of the body • Improves the balance and posture • Improves coordination
Restorative asanas or yoga poses		
Basic Relaxation pose	NA	• Lowers blood pressure • Slows heart rate • Releases muscular tension • Reduces fatigue • Improves sleep • Enhances immune response • Helps to manage chronic pain • Quiets the frontal lobes of the brain
Cat Cow (Restorative, upright version)	Cat: Marjariasana Cow: Bitilasana Cat Cow: Chakravakasana	• Awakens the spine • Energizes, due to the back extension • Improves sitting and standing posture • Enhances coordination • Stretches and strengthens the front and back of the body • Reduces back pain
Corpse pose	Savasana	• Reduces blood pressure • Calms the mind • Enhances relaxation throughout the body • Reduces headache • Decreases fatigue • Decreases insomnia
Queen's pose	Salamba Baddha Konasana	• Opens the back • Opens the pelvic region

Reclining Twist with a Bolster	NA	• Reduces strain in the back • Reduces strain in the intercostal muscles • As the muscles relax, breathing is enhanced
Restorative Child's pose on bolsters	Restorative Balasana	• Engages the parasympathetic nervous system and encourages the relaxation response • Reduces strain in the neck, back, and hips, and calms the mind • Helps relieve anxiety, stress, and fatigue
Seated Bound Angle pose	Baddha Konasana	• Opens the hips • Opens the pelvis • Lowers blood pressure • Helps with breathing problems
Side Resting pose with bolster	NA	• Reduces fatigue • Stimulates the abdominal organs • Enhances relaxation in the nervous system • Decreases blood pressure
Supported Reclining Bound Angle pose	Supta Baddha Konasana	• Opens the chest • Opens the abdomen • Opens the pelvis • Lowers blood pressure • Helps with breathing problems
Supported Wide-Angle Seated Forward Fold	Upavistha Konasana	• Quiets the organs of digestion and elimination
Mudras or hand postures		
NA	Adi Mudra	• Improves sleep (and reduces snoring) • Increases lung capacity • Improves the flow of oxygen to the brain • Relaxes the nervous system
NA	Anjali Mudra	• Balances and unites the right and left sides of the body, physically, emotionally, and mentally
NA	Apana Mudra	• Eliminates waste from the body, as well as enhances mental or physical digestion • Reduces constipation and increases the regularity of bowel movements • Increases urination and sweating
NA	Apana Vayu Mudra	• Helps heart-related issues such as high blood pressure, palpitations, and arteriosclerosis • Helps gastrointestinal issues, including heartburn and indigestion

Selected pranayama and yoga poses	Sanskrit name	Perceived benefits
NA	Brahma (or Purna) Mudra	• Releases blocked energy and releases this energy to the brain • Calms the mind • Enhances relaxation • Releases negative energies • Thought to bring the individual to a higher meditative state
NA	Buddhi Mudra	• Enhances intuitive communication and intuitive knowledge • Develops intuition • Provides relief from a number of ailments, including digestive issues, skin disorders, blood-related diseases, and blood and kidney disorders
NA	Chinmaya Mudra	• Improves digestion and enhances the flow of energy in the body, particularly in the thoracic region of the spine • Promotes breathing in the lungs
NA	Dhyana Mudra	• Promotes a calming energy • Clarifies thought • Decreases ego involvement • Brings peace
NA	Ganesha Mudra	• Removes obstacles from life • Enhances feelings of positivity and bravery in the face of difficult issues
NA	Gyan or Chin Mudra	• Improves concentration • Stimulates the brain • Strengthens the nervous system • Increases feelings of relaxation and stress reduction • Enhances sleep • Increases energy • Improves focus • Reduces lower back pain
NA	Prana Mudra	• Increases feelings of energy and strength • Decreases feelings of fatigue • Reduces stress • Improves sleep • Reduces blood pressure • Increases immunity • Decreases acidity and ulcers in the gut • Decreases inflammation in the body

NA	Shuni Mudra	• Enhances feelings of patience, discipline, and stability • Helps to bring focus and discipline
NA	Survya Ravi Mudra	• Enhances feelings of balance • Enhances physical and spiritual well-being
NA	Vayu Mudra	• Improves high blood pressure • Reduces abdominal discomfort, bloating, and other air-related conditions • Improves health and decreases pain and issues from conditions including arthritis, gout, and sciatica

Tips of the Trade from the Pros

We surveyed hundreds of people from around the world to find out who is using yoga and how they are using it in practice. We learned a tremendous amount of information from the many providers who are using yoga for clients with stroke.

Who Is Using Yoga in Practice?

We learned that occupational therapists, recreational therapists, physical therapists, counselors, and yoga therapists are the clinicians most often using yoga for clients with stroke. Based on the survey, yoga is most commonly used in outpatient rehabilitation clinics. Approximately 50% of the clinicians using yoga in practice who completed the survey were trained yoga instructors, teachers, or therapists. The rest of the survey participants learned about using yoga through their own personal practice, education, or continuing education. Importantly, about 95% of the survey participants reported that they had a personal yoga practice.

How Do Therapists Introduce the Idea of Yoga to a Therapy Session or the Clinical Setting?

We asked the therapists how they introduce yoga to a new client. Some therapists talked about yoga as yoga and used the English or Sanskrit names of postures when describing it. However, most therapists indicated that they introduced yoga as yoga to some potential clients, but for others they talked about yoga as being part of the therapy or intervention or as a way to promote relaxation and help with sleep. For many therapists, it "depended" on the client; sometimes the therapist introduced the intervention as yoga but sometimes as an exercise for breathing or balance. For other therapists, it also depended on the facility where they were working. It appears that some facilities or therapy managers were more open to the idea of using yoga as part of clinical practice than others.

As one recreational therapist who worked in long-term care said:

> It's really very successful with the vast majority of our residents. I think…because of the ease of some of the moves in yoga, so if I'm just being able to focus on my breath and not having to…be too self-conscious about your physical ability or limitations. You know, or even the range of motion, it really can branch across all of our clients. With that in mind you really can really have such an emphasis on the range of your movement which has been very popular with our residents with multiple sclerosis who are experiencing like a continual loss of function. So it's something they connected to and stay motivated with when other exercise programs kind of lose a bit of, they lose motivation because of their declining ability.

How to Document the Use of Yoga

We included questions in the survey about documentation of yoga for insurance purposes. Most yoga or rehabilitation therapists did have to document the intervention in some way. We also chatted with some managers of rehabilitation groups or clinics to talk about the documentation of yoga as an intervention during typical stroke rehabilitation. Some clients with stroke may pay out of pocket for yoga therapy; however, many will be reliant on insurance to pay for post-stroke therapies. Therefore, yoga may be offered by rehabilitation therapists or counselors during regular post-stroke scheduled therapies, and therapists told us they are documenting the use of yoga in different ways. It appears that some therapists used yoga as a "modality" or a part of treatment versus providing an entire session of yoga. This is likely related to the clinician type (yoga therapist versus recreational or occupational therapist) and the setting (acute rehabilitation or outpatient rehabilitation versus a yoga therapist providing yoga in a private office). It appears that documentation is also somewhat based on the use of insurance for payment or the type of insurance that is available.

Some tips for documentation of yoga for insurance reasons are given below.

- In the United States, Medicare will not pay for group yoga sessions, but some private insurance companies will allow for some group intervention time. Depending on the facility, this may allow for group yoga, and the social aspect of yoga may be helpful to some people with stroke. A yoga group allows for support from others and the clients often encourage others to continue to attend yoga or to progress in the yoga postures.

- Many yoga or rehabilitation therapists included yoga under specific words or codes in the documentation. Examples include:

  - therapeutic exercise

  - therapeutic activities

  - neuromuscular control exercise

  - neuro re-education

  - patient or family education

  - dynamic balance or postural control

  - activity linked to functional tasks

  - description of the movement or the pose (but not the name of the yoga pose)

  - use of or engagement in leisure activities

  - physical benefits of the postures, education, and breathing

  - intervention for mental health symptoms

  - as a coping mechanism used in mental health but also for people going through painful or stressful physical interventions or testing (i.e. MRI, painful stretching) after the stroke

  - use of a physical intervention for weight bearing, balance, strengthening, gross motor control, or other needs that are typically addressed during the rehabilitation process after stroke

  - core strength to increase the ability to transfer (to the toilet, to the tub bench, to the car)

  - stress management.

When asked for an example of documenting the use of yoga, one occupational therapist stated:

It depends what I am targeting—"range of motion therapeutic exercise completed with coordinated breath and movement," or that I addressed anxiety with mind-body interventions including x, y, z… I typically do not type or document the word yoga unless the patient identifies yoga as a preferred occupation.

A physical therapist stated: "Patient participated in standing balance activity with standby or contact guard assist for three minutes with no loss of balance noted."

- Other therapists included the words yoga or yoga practices in the documentation after stroke. Examples include:

  - breathing exercises with meaningful movements

  - modified or adapted yoga for multiple and different reasons

  - specific names of postures; some therapists included the Sanskrit names of the poses as well

  - specific names of the asana and/or pranayama and the clinical rationale for the inclusion in the therapy session.

Tips to Develop Community-Based Yoga Sites for People with Disabilities

We hope that this book helps to create more accessible yoga opportunities in the community and for people with disabilities. We talked with two individuals about how they are currently involved in developing accessible yoga programming in their communities. While these reports about providing adaptive yoga in the community are not specific to serving clients with stroke, we hope that much of the information is relevant to attempting to build a larger adaptive yoga community.

Torrey is an Assistant Studio Manager at Meraki Yoga in Fort Collins, CO (https://meraki yogastudio.com). Meraki Yoga donated space for our photo shoot with Betty and has recently begun to develop some community-based yoga programming for individuals with disabilities. In her own words, Torrey tells us about herself and answers our questions.

Can you tell us more about how you came to the decision to begin working with clients with disabilities and providing them yoga? Or why? Is it related to your background? To your interests? To your yoga or clinical training?

So, I am actually not a certified yoga instructor. I work at Meraki Yoga as a Brand Ambassador and Assistant Studio Manager. My decision to have this event came from a combination of my love for yoga along with my passion for helping individuals with special needs and/or disabilities. I graduated in 2016 with a Bachelor of Arts degree in Psychology with an emphasis in Family and Child Development. Upon completion of my undergraduate degree, I earned a Post-Baccalaureate Certificate in Communication Sciences and Disorders. I have recently submitted graduate school applications, in which I hope to earn my Master of Science Degree in Speech-Language Pathology.

In October of 2017 I began volunteering at Speech and Language Stimulation Center with Annie, a certified speech-language pathologist. It was during a session with Annie's 42-year-old client with cerebral palsy that I had the idea to plan this particular event. In the middle of the session Annie noticed that her client's muscles were especially tight, so she began to work her clenched arms down to a more relaxed position, and while doing so, kind of offhandedly said, "You need yoga!" It was then that a lightbulb went off in my head! "How amazing would it be to hold an event partnering these two companies (Meraki Yoga and Speech and Language Stimulation Center) and bring two things together that I am so passionate about." I later proposed the idea to the owners of Meraki Yoga and they were instantly on board and loved the idea! Since planning the event I have become even more passionate about providing events and outings for individuals with special needs, as I feel that there are not a lot of opportunities like this in the community. I am hoping for a great turnout for this event, so much so that we decided to hold a second one in the summer or early fall!

What populations with disabilities are you trying to serve?

We really are wanting to serve all populations. At this event we will offer two different yoga classes. One will be designed for children with disabilities, ages 4 years to 13 years old. This class will be imaginative and playful and will combine simple yoga poses with engaging songs and stories that exercise social, sensory, and motor skills.

The second class will be designed for adults, wheelchair users, and/or less physically mobile clients. This class will include active and restorative yoga poses that target the fifth chakra, our communication center, while incorporating breathing exercises that help relieve stress and anxiety, as well as to improve concentration and focus.

For both classes we will have licensed occupational therapists and physical therapists to provide support, assists, and modifications.

What have been some challenges in getting adapted or accessible yoga to your studio or to your community?

I think the biggest challenge has just been the marketing aspect of it. It has been kind of difficult finding places to pass out flyers and places that will actually encourage people to sign up for the event! So I guess I am just nervous that we won't have as great of a turnout that I am hoping for.

What has been the response to adapted or accessible yoga at your studio or in your community?

The response at our studio and in our community has been very positive! The community of students and instructors at Meraki Yoga has been very supportive and excited to see adapted and/or accessible yoga at our studio.

Are you or other individuals a yoga therapist (versus a yoga teacher) or are you a different kind of therapist (occupational, recreational, physical therapist)? Tell us a little about your background.

> As I previously mentioned, I am not a certified yoga instructor. Although, I am becoming more and more interested in becoming a certified yoga instructor to specifically teach yoga to individuals with special needs and/or disabilities. Whether I incorporate yoga into my practice and profession as a future speech-language pathologist, start an event planning business centered around adapted and/or accessible yoga events, or open a studio where the main focus is inclusive yoga, I am certain that I want to work in this field in some way.
>
> The yoga instructor who will be teaching both classes at our event is a licensed physician's assistant in addition to being a certified yoga instructor.

Please tell us about suggestions you have to help other yoga teachers or therapists who want to make yoga more accessible in their community.

> Taking on an event like this can definitely be challenging, specifically when it comes to working all of the pieces together and trying to get enough people to volunteer and participate. But, my advice for anyone who is interested in making yoga more accessible in their community is to find volunteers who have a background in occupational therapy, physical therapy, speech therapy, etc. and who are passionate about the benefits of yoga for individuals with special needs and/or disabilities. Lastly, if anyone is interested in this field, I would just say that the most important thing is to put your whole heart and positive energy into it because you'll be providing a service to people who do not have these services readily available to them and they will be so grateful for it!

Jennifer Jayanti Atkins is a 500-hour-level certified yoga teacher, also in Fort Collins, CO. Jennifer has been teaching yoga for clients with Parkinson's Disease, multiple sclerosis, and traumatic brain injury. Her website is at https://jayantiyoga.com. Many of the yoga classes she teaches are supported through the city, allowing individuals to attend the yoga for a very reduced rate. In her own words, Jennifer answers some of our questions about adaptive yoga in the community.

Can you tell us more about how you came to the decision to begin working with clients with disabilities and providing them yoga? Or why? Is it related to your background? To your interests? To your yoga or clinical training?

> I suppose my reasons are from my background in education in kinesiology, and even more so from my original yoga teacher training at Kripalu Center for Yoga and Health. The Kripalu yoga tradition is known as the "yoga of compassion" and I absorbed this deeply in my early trainings. I did not realize I had an interest or ability in adaptive yoga until the opportunity presented itself. Really "right place, right time, with the right skills, and an open heart."

What populations with disabilities are you trying to serve?

I have been serving people with Parkinson's Disease for 4.5 years, people with multiple sclerosis for 2.5 years, and people with traumatic brain injuries for the last year. This is accomplished through ongoing group classes in the city of Fort Collins and visiting some individuals in their homes throughout northern Colorado.

What have been some challenges in getting adapted or accessible yoga to your studio or to your community?

I have been so fortunate in my profession thus far. I have had nothing but support and success in developing and facilitating my adaptive yoga programs in this community. My classes are held in the large yoga studio within Raintree Athletic Club (a local fitness center). The club is very accessible and the management is accommodating. They are quite happy to be contributing to the community in this way, and being a team member with them for seven years, they give me total freedom and responsibility to oversee and conduct my adaptive yoga classes. I should add, the population I serve are no longer working and most individuals are on disability. This allowed me to conduct my classes in the mid-afternoon hours when regular yoga classes at the fitness center are not usually held. These are ideal times for my clients. If I were trying to serve a population that was still working, this would likely be my biggest challenge—finding appropriate, accessible studio space, at a time that isn't already serving the "typical" population.

What has been the response to adapted or accessible yoga at your studio or in your community?

The response has been overwhelmingly positive on all counts. My yoga for Parkinson's Disease classes have increased from two classes a week to three classes a week. Yoga for multiple sclerosis has increased from one class a week to twice a week. The yoga for traumatic brain injury classes are taking off with requests for more in the year ahead. Class sizes can be quite large (between 12 and 25 individuals) and hold strong with dedicated student attendance and with new folks joining all of the time.

Are you or other individuals a yoga therapist (versus a yoga teacher) or are you a different kind of therapist (occupational, recreational, physical therapist)? Tell us a little about your background.

I consider myself an Adaptive Yoga Specialist. I am a certified yoga instructor of 19 years, highly experienced and skilled with advanced training credentials.

Please tell us about suggestions you have to help other yoga teachers or therapists who want to make yoga more accessible in their community.

To hold safe and effective yoga classes not only requires an experienced and compassionate teacher, but also *props, lots* of *props*! Required for every student in the yoga classes: sturdy chairs without wheels, mats, firm bolsters, foam blocks, blankets. Other props that are optional but highly recommended include: yoga sand bags, fit falls, broom sticks or bamboo poles. The building and the room must be accessible, ideally with adjoining accessible bathrooms. Also, I try to have several assistants in class, sometimes students from the Colorado State University Occupational Therapy program. Assistants are necessary not only for setting the room up with all of the necessary props, but also to assist individuals as needed during the yoga intervention, to best maintain safety.

Yoga May Be Good for the Caregiver Too!

You may notice that the family and friends of the client with stroke are often around and helpful and often are feeling quite stressed. Caregivers may sustain high levels of stress and worry after their loved one sustains a stroke. Family and friends who provide care are considered to be informal caregivers, not paid or formal caregivers. These informal caregivers are vital to the client's progress, recovery, education, and living situation (for example, going home versus going to a nursing home or independent living center). However, the informal caregiver needs to take care of themselves and promote their own health and wellness. The stress of caregiving may negatively impact the emotional, mental, and physical health of the informal caregiver. Caregivers, particularly female caregivers, are more likely to give up their leisure and health-promoting activities in order to provide care. Caregivers are also likely to be exhausted by the time their family member gets home from the hospital, because the caregiver has spent so much time at home with their loved one. The paradox of this is, of course, that the caregiver will need that energy when their loved one comes home. For this reason, and many more, teaching the caregiver ways to take care of themselves during the stroke recovery process may benefit the person who has had a stroke, because the caregiver will be able to be more present, and benefit the caregiver, because of the health-related benefits associated with yoga.

Due to the stresses of informal caregiving, there are great guides online to help family and friends who are caregivers after a stroke (see www.stroke.org/we-can-help/caregivers-and-family/careliving-guide). Additionally, we also recommend including the caregiver in the yoga sessions when appropriate. Yoga, as a part of rehabilitation during the acute or chronic phases of stroke, may be a shared activity between the caregiver and the client with stroke. Having a shared activity may decrease the stress of caregiving and positively influence the shared relationship between the two people involved.

We always invite caregivers to attend the yoga sessions during our yoga studies. Sometimes the caregivers choose to use the time to read a book or go grocery shopping, but often they choose to attend yoga. There appears to be many benefits of including the caregiver in the yoga sessions. For example, we have found that:

- yoga may help reduce the stress and worry that the caregiver is feeling

- yoga may improve physical strength, range of motion, or flexibility for the caregiver, allowing them to be able to better provide physical care (like transfers or dressing) while at the same time decreasing the risk of injury related to caregiving

- yoga allows the caregiver time to be in the moment and take care of themselves

- when joining us, the caregiver knows that their loved one is safe and well taken care of, allowing the caregiver to really engage in and enjoy the yoga

- caregivers who attended eight weeks of classes during one stroke and yoga and occupational therapy study benefited from a 47% decrease in caregiver burden (Hinsey, *et al.*, 2015)

- attending yoga with their loved one may help the caregiver realize how much the client with stroke can actually do

- if the client with stroke has aphasia or other post-stroke communication issues, attending yoga with their loved one may help the caregiver learn how to communicate more effectively, using short instructions and giving time to process the information

- doing the yoga together may help improve attendance to yoga and adherence or compliance with home-based yoga programming

- yoga improves the strength and flexibility in caregivers, which can help them provide more physical care, if needed, for their loved one.

Select Book Resources
Asanas, Pranayama, or Meditation

- Bhajan, Y. (1974). *Kundalini Yoga Sadhana Guidelines* (2nd Ed). Espanola, NM: Kundalini Research Institute.

- Hanson, R. (2009). *Buddha's Brain: The Practical Neuroscience of Happiness, Love, and Wisdom.* Oakland, CA: New Harbinger Publications.

- McGonigal, K. (2009). *Yoga for Pain Relief: Simple Practices to Calm Your Mind and Heal Your Chronic Pain.* Oakland, CA: New Harbinger Publications.

- Prinster, T. (2014). *Yoga for Cancer: A Guide to Managing Side Effects, Boosting Immunity, and Improving Recovery for Cancer Survivors.* New York: Simon and Schuster.

- Shaw, S. (2003). *The Little Book of Yoga Breathing: Pranayama Made Easy...* San Francisco, CA: Weiser Books.

Restorative Yoga

- Flamm, S. (2013). *Restorative Yoga with Assists: A Manual for Teachers and Students of Yoga* (2nd Ed). Self-published.

- Grossman, G. B. (2015). *Restorative Yoga for Life: A Relaxing Way to De-Stress, Re-Energize, and Find Balance.* Avon, MA: Adams Media.

- Rentz, K. (2005). *Yoganap: Relaxation Poses for Deep Relaxation.* Cambridge, MA: Da Capo Press.

Yoga Philosophy

- Iyengar, B. (1965). *Light on Yoga.* New York: Schocken Books.

- Mishra, R. S. (1972). *The Textbook of Yoga Psychology: A New Translation and Interpretation of Patanjali's Yoga Sutras for Meaningful Application in All Modern Psychologic Disciplines.* London: Lyrebird Press Ltd.

Internet Resources

- Our website: www.mergingyogaandrehabilitation.com

- 3HO: Healthy, Happy, Holy Organization: Resources for Kundalini Yoga: www.3ho.org/kundalini-yoga

- International Association of Yoga Therapists: www.iayt.org

- Yoga International: www.yogainternational.com

- Yoga Journal: www.yogajournal.com

CHAPTER 14

Prevention of Future Strokes and Injuries

In this chapter, we review the risk factors for future strokes, and how yoga may help to reduce the seven primary risk factors for recurrent strokes. We also provide specific tips for therapists about areas to focus on that may help to reduce yoga-related injuries when working with individuals who are post-stroke.

Preventing Future Strokes: The Role of Yoga

According to the National Stroke Association (2018) in the United States, for individuals who have had a stroke, there is a 25–35% chance of a recurrent stroke, and the risk for a second stroke within the first five years is more than 40%. Even more alarming is that 80% of recurrent strokes could be prevented through changes in lifestyle and through interventions (National Stroke Association). Importantly, yoga may play a part in the prevention of future strokes. Below, each of the seven primary risk factors for a second stroke are identified, as is the possible link to yoga.

- **High blood pressure**: Uncontrolled high blood pressure has been shown to double or quadruple an individual's risk for a stroke. Lifestyle changes, such as reducing sodium in the diet, reducing the intake of high-cholesterol foods, eating fruits and vegetables, and quitting smoking, are well known to reduce blood pressure. The recommendation of getting at least 30 minutes of physical activity per day is also known to reduce blood pressure. A review of the yoga literature identified that yoga reduces blood pressure in individuals with hypertension, as well as reducing other stroke risk factors, including reductions in cholesterol and body weight (Okonta, 2012).

- **Increased weight**: Obesity, and its co-morbidities and complications (such as diabetes or high blood pressure), increase the risk of a stroke. Diet modifications are one way to reduce weight, and another is through physical activity. Yoga, of course, is considered a physical activity, and a number of research studies have indicated that yoga is associated with weight loss, including a study that identified that a regular yoga practice was associated with weight maintenance or loss in individuals who were overweight

(Kristal, *et al.*, 2005). These findings indicate that yoga may be a good tool to help with weight maintenance or loss.

- **Sedentary lifestyle**: Recommendations exist that suggest that in order to reduce the threat of another stroke, an individual should aim for 30 minutes per day of physical activity. A 30-minute yoga practice every day is an achievable goal and could be implemented in therapy or on one's own. Yoga can also be used to augment physical activity, because the stretching that occurs during yoga can nicely complement other physical activities, such as walking, running, or biking. Yoga is ubiquitously described as helping the body feel much better, and its adaptability to every age and type of ability level makes it really accessible.

- **Alcohol intake**: The National Institute on Alcohol Abuse and Alcoholism (2018) has identified that more than seven drinks per week for women, and 14 drinks per week for men, is considered excessive. What does yoga have to do with drinking in moderation or not at all? The answer may not be obvious at first, but there is a small amount of yoga research that indicates that yoga may help to reduce dependence on alcohol (Reddy, *et al.*, 2014) or the amount of daily alcoholic drinks (Hallgren, *et al.*, 2014).

- **Atrial fibrillation**: Atrial fibrillation is a rapid and irregular heart rate. It can lead to many heart-related complications, including stroke, blood clots, and heart failure (American Heart Association, 2017). While typical treatment for atrial fibrillation is medication, yoga has been shown to treat atrial fibrillation also! Researchers worked with clients with paroxysmal atrial fibrillation (individuals whose heartbeat returned to normal within seven days, with or without treatment) and provided two 60-minute yoga sessions for three months. Yoga was found to reduce symptomatic atrial fibrillation episodes, symptomatic non-atrial fibrillation episodes, and asymptomatic atrial fibrillation episodes (Lakkireddy, *et al.*, 2013).

- **Diabetes**: Primary methods to manage and treat diabetes are intentional dietary choices, exercise, and sometimes medicine. Yoga has been shown to treat diabetes, with the most research evidence available for treating Type 2 Diabetes Mellitus. A systematic review of 25 studies of yoga for people with Type 2 Diabetes Mellitus found that there were reductions in a number of risk indices, including improved: glucose tolerance, insulin sensitivity, cholesterol and blood lipids, weight, body mass index, body composition, systolic and diastolic blood pressure, and oxidative stress. This review also suggested that reducing stress, decreasing the activation/reactivity of the sympathoadrenal system, and vagal stimulation may be the initial pathways to decreasing risk for Type 2 Diabetes Mellitus and its associated complications (Innes and Vincent, 2007).

- **Smoking**: Typical approaches to quitting smoking include specific aids such as nicotine patches or pills, medicine, and counseling. In addition to, or instead of, these approaches, yoga has been shown to assist in quitting smoking. For example, women in a research study that compared cognitive behavioral therapy plus yoga to a general health and wellness program had higher levels of abstinence in the yoga group, and this lasted through six months following the intervention (Bock, *et al.*, 2012). These researchers demonstrated that yoga was an effective complement to cognitive behavioral therapy in terms of abstinence from smoking.

Taken all together, there is substantial evidence that yoga can help to reduce or manage the risk factors for a recurrent stroke. This is particularly important when working with your client during the "teachable moment" that may occur after a stroke. The teachable moment is that period of time following a scary or momentous health event, such as a stroke, when people are most likely to make changes to their lifestyle in order to prevent the reoccurrence of the health event. Hopefully, seeing the vast health-related benefits of participating in a regular yoga practice will be enough reason for your client to participate in yoga with you and on their own after discharge from your care. If not, we hope that this included information and the vast literature on the benefits of yoga for addressing the primary risk factors for a recurrent stroke may speak to your client.

Preventing Injuries in Individuals Who Are Post-Stroke: The Role of the Therapist

While injuries are unlikely during yoga, there are considerations for the yoga or rehabilitation therapist to pay attention to when working with someone post-stroke. A stroke may cause reduced recognition of feelings of pain, temperature, pain, or sharpness on the hemiplegic side of the body. This could inadvertently cause or allow for an injury if the limbs or body are not attended to. Therefore, the therapist should pay attention to the following issues.

- **The placement of the limbs during yoga**: Visually evaluate the individual's body for unnatural positioning. The individual who is post-stroke may not be able to evaluate comfort or pain. Ensure that upper and lower extremities are placed away from moving parts (such as the wheels or spokes of a wheelchair). Also ensure that proper wheelchair seating is used, and apply these techniques to chairs if they are being used in yoga.

- **The hemiplegic hand**: If the hand or fist is clenched, make sure that the fingernails are not cutting into the hand. Hemiplegic hands, wrists, and fingers may be in a resting hand splint, and the fingers should be stretched. Yoga provides a great opportunity for the stretching of the hemiplegic hand; therapists are encouraged to co-treat with a therapist who uses hand-stretching modalities as appropriate.

- **Correct use of durable medical equipment**: Use appropriate support surfaces for transfers or to support the affected limb or side.

- **Reduce moisture**: Moisture may lead to skin breakdowns, so the therapist should monitor drooling, enuresis (accidental urination), and other fluids to ensure that there is no pooling of moisture during the yoga session. Note: Moisture can also pool in the clenched hand, so care should be taken to ensure that the moisture is dried off as needed.

- **Ankle plantarflexion contractures**: After a stroke, an individual may have impaired gait quality, potentially due to a contracture in the ankle plantarflexor muscle. When this happens, the client will have "foot drop" and will have pointed toes. Foot drop causes great problems with walking and transferring. Some individuals may use an ankle foot orthosis to help prevent or manage an ankle contracture. During yoga, these ankle foot orthoses may be removed to work on ankle range of motion; however, it is important that the client or the therapist correctly reapply the orthosis after yoga. Therapists should be trained in the proper application of the ankle foot orthosis to avoid injury, including skin ulcers/wounds.

- **Painful shoulders** occur in up to 25% of people following stroke. The American Stroke Association (Winstein, *et al.*, 2016) identified that hemiplegic shoulder pain may have a variety of origins and has some connection with complex regional pain syndrome. To address shoulder pain broadly, it is recommended to use proper positioning techniques and maintain shoulder range of motion—both of which can be addressed in yoga.

  - A subluxed shoulder (or, more technically, a glenohumeral subluxation) is a dislocation of the shoulder (specifically, the humeral head slips out of the glenoid cavity) caused by the weight of the affected hemiplegic arm. Subluxation may also be caused by the muscles being too weak to hold the bone in place, or, when the arm is flaccid in a hemiparetic state, the tissue may be stretched too far by gravity or the improper handling of the arm (i.e. the arm is pulled on by caregivers during transfers). Thus, it is essential that therapists understand how to transfer individuals with a hemiplegic arm so as not to cause further harm. Proper seating positioning is also important, and therapists may want to provide a pillow for support when the person is engaged in seated yoga.

  - Frozen shoulders. A frozen shoulder is characterized by pain and stiffness. Frozen shoulders are also common in people who are post-stroke, because of the lack of use of the shoulder on the hemiplegic side. In order to prevent a frozen shoulder, the therapist should:

    » attend to the positioning and support of the affected arm

> » help the individual with their range of motion by encouraging use of the affected size or using passive range of motion techniques to encourage movement. Yoga may be a great addition to therapy to decrease the development of a frozen shoulder

> » recognize when the individual has reached their limit of exercise for the day.

- **Swelling**: Swelling may also be an issue in the extremities for the hemiparetic side of the body, due to periods of no or little movement or if the arm is held down to the side of the body (gravity causes fluids to pool). Swelling is problematic for the individual who is post-stroke because it can cause pressure sores due to the reduced blood flow in the limb. Swelling also limits full range of motion in the limb, which leads to contractures or stiffening of the joint. Finally, swelling is uncomfortable and can be painful in the area around the swollen tissues. In order to prevent or reduce swelling, the therapist can:

  - ensure that the affected limb is elevated; arms or legs that hang down are much more prone to swelling

  - incorporate therapeutic massage into yoga to move the fluid out of the limb

  - ensure that the individual is wearing any prescribed compression stockings during yoga

  - include yoga poses that encourage movement of the limbs above the heart, such as Five Pointed Star (Utthita Tadasana), Chair (Utkatasana), and Warrior I and II (Virabhadrasana I and II). These postures are described in Chapter 6.

- **Unexpected behavior**: Following a stroke, the client's behavior may be more impulsive and less cautious, due to the location of the stroke in the brain. Therefore, it is important that the therapist pays attention to safety and monitors for impulsive behaviors. A stroke on the right side of the brain (resulting in left-sided impairments) may lead to changes in behavior, including the denial of disability. In these individuals, frequent reminders of ability or disability may be needed.

- **Visual changes**: As identified in Chapter 2, visual changes such as homonymous hemianopsia (inability to see half of the visual field, usually the right or left), diplopia (double vision), and quadrantanopia (inability to see upper or lower quadrants of the visual field) may interfere with the individual's ability to see dangers in front of them. Therefore, it is important for the therapist to provide verbal cues and demonstrations, as well as to monitor the area for any objects that may cause harm.

- **Fall prevention**: Falls are more likely after stroke due to impairments in gait and balance, and individuals who are post-stroke are more likely to break the hip or pelvis during a fall than older adults who are not post-stroke (Truelsen, *et al.*, 2006). Falls also lead to a fear of falling, which in turn has a substantial negative cascade of events, including reduced engagement in life activities (Schmid and Rittman, 2007, 2009). During yoga, there are options to do the practice from a chair, standing, or supine on the floor or mat table. When progressing your client to a standing position, use care to ensure that there are safety measures in place in case of unexpected loss of balance.

- **A gait belt is not a yoga strap**: In Chapter 6 there is substantial mention of the use of a gait belt instead of a yoga strap. It is perfectly acceptable to use a gait belt instead of a yoga strap to extend the reach or make a posture more accessible for an individual. However, it is not acceptable to use a yoga strap instead of a gait belt for transfers. A yoga strap does not have the same level of durability or strength and should not be used instead of a gait belt.

- **Extra time for processing**: As detailed in Chapter 2, substantial cognitive changes may happen for individuals who are post-stroke. It is important to remember that individuals may need extra time to process information, including in an emergency situation.

Finally, in our research, we have shown that inattention to detail and inattention to the physical body may contribute to post-stroke falls (Schmid, *et al.*, 2013b). Therefore, improvements in the physical body and mind-body connection may lead to other improvements such as reduced fall rates and improved physical activity. For example, participating in yoga may lead to improvements in mindfulness, body responsiveness, and the ability to better manage constraints to fuller participation in life, all of which may lead to additional physiological and psychological improvements (Van Puymbroeck, Smith, and Schmid, 2011; Van Puymbroeck, Schmid, *et al.*, 2011; Van Puymbroeck, *et al.*, 2014). We have also found that participating in yoga helps reduce perceived activity constraints, allowing people to increase engagement in enjoyable life activities (Van Puymbroeck, Smith, and Schmid, 2011; Van Puymbroeck, Schmid, *et al.*, 2011).

Being a yoga or rehabilitation therapist for an individual who is post-stroke can be highly rewarding. But, therapy also requires substantial attention to detail and nuances of care so that the individual is treated in a manner that will minimize additional injury. Attending to these details is important, and, while it may seem overwhelming initially, it becomes second nature after a while!

References

3HO (2018). Mudra. Accessed on 7/23/18 at https://www.3ho.org/kundalini-yoga/mudra.

Altenburger, P., Schmid, A., Van Puymbroeck, V., and Miller, K. (2016). Impact of yoga on postural stability in stroke. *International Journal of Neurorehabilitation, 3*(1), 195.

American Heart Association. (2017). What is atrial fibrillation (AFib or AF)? Accessed on 09/05/2018 at www.heart.org/HEARTORG/Conditions/Arrhythmia/AboutArrhythmia/What-is-Atrial-Fibrillation-AFib-or-AF_UCM_423748_Article.jsp.

American Stroke Association. (2016). Impact of stroke (stroke statistics). Accessed on 09/05/2018 at www.strokeassociation.org/STROKEORG/AboutStroke/Impact-of-Stroke-Stroke-statistics_UCM_310728_Article.jsp#.WusfL2bMzOQ.

American Stroke Association. (2017). Ischemic strokes (clots). Accessed on 09/05/2018 at www.strokeassociation.org/STROKEORG/AboutStroke/TypesofStroke/IschemicClots/Ischemic-Strokes-Clots_UCM_310939_Article.jsp#.Wusd7WbMyi5.

Atler, K., Portz, J. D., Van Puymbroeck, M., and Schmid, A. (2017). Outcomes of a multimodal group self-management intervention for fall prevention: Qualitative perspectives on MY-OT among people post stroke. *British Journal of Occupational Therapy, 8*(5), 155–162.

Australian Stroke Association. (2018). Vision loss after stroke fact sheet. Accessed on 15/04/2018 at https://strokefoundation.org.au/About-Stroke/Help-after-stroke/Stroke-resources-and-fact-sheets/Vision-loss-after-stroke-fact-sheet.

Bastille, J. V., and Gill-Body, K. M. (2004). A yoga-based exercise program for people with chronic poststroke hemiparesis. *Physical Therapy, 84*(1), 33–48.

Bell, B. (2007). Yoga for stroke survivors. *Yoga Journal*, August 28, 2007.

Berg, K., Wood-Dauphinee, S., and Williams, J. I. (1995). The Balance Scale: Reliability assessment with elderly residents and patients with an acute stroke. *Scandinavian Journal of Rehabilitation Medicine, 27*(1), 27–36.

Bhajan, Y. (1974). *Kundalini Yoga Sadhana Guidelines* (2nd Ed). Espanola, NM: Kundalini Research Institute.

Black, D. S., Cole, S., Irwin, M. R., Breen, E., *et al.* (2013). Yogic meditation reverses NF-KB and IRF-related transcriptome dynamics in leukocytes of family dementia caregivers in a randomized controlled trial. *Psychoneuroendocrinology, 38*(3), 348–355.

Bock, B. C., Fava, J. L., Gaskins, R., Morrow, K. M., *et al.* (2012). Yoga as a complementary treatment for smoking cessation in women. *Journal of Women's Health, 21*(2), 240–248.

Botner, E. M., Miller, W. C., and Eng, J. J. (2005). Measurement properties of the Activities-specific Balance Confidence Scale among individuals with stroke. *Disability and Rehabilitation, 27*(4), 156–163.

Campbell Burton, C., Murray, J., Holmes, J., Astin, F., Greenwood, D., and Knapp, P. (2013). Frequency of anxiety after stroke: A systematic review and meta-analysis of observational studies. *International Journal of Stroke, 8*(7), 545–559.

Carey, J. R., Kimberley, T. J., Lewis, S. M., Auerbach, E. J., *et al.* (2002). Analysis of fMRI and finger tracking training in subjects with chronic stroke. *Brain, 125*(Pt 4), 773–788.

Chan, W., Immink, M. A., and Hillier, S. (2012). Yoga and exercise for symptoms of depression and anxiety in people with poststroke disability: A randomized, controlled pilot trial. *Alternative Therapies in Health and Medicine, 18*(3), 34–43.

Chiacchiero, M., Dresely, B., Silva, U., DeLosReyes, R., and Vorik, B. (2010). The relationship between range of movement, flexibility, and balance in the elderly. *Topics in Geriatric Rehabilitation, 26*(2), 148–155.

Cramer, H., Lauche, R., Langhorst, J., and Dobos, G. (2013). Yoga for depression: A systematic review and meta-analysis. *Depression and Anxiety, 30*(11), 1068–1083.

Crowe, B. M., Van Puymbroeck, M., and Schmid, A. A. (2016). Yoga as coping: A conceptual framework for meaningful participation in yoga. *International Journal of Yoga Therapy, 26*(1), 123–129.

Desveaux, L., Lee, A., Goldstein, R., and Brooks, D. (2015). Yoga in the management of chronic disease: A systematic review and meta-analysis. *Medical Care, 53*(7), 653–661.

Donnelly, K. Z., Linnea, K., Grant, D. A., and Lichtenstein, J. (2017). The feasibility and impact of a yoga pilot programme on the quality-of-life of adults with acquired brain injury. *Brain Injury, 31*(2), 208–214.

Flamm, S. (2013). *Restorative Yoga with Assists: A Manual for Teachers and Students of Yoga* (2nd Ed). Self-published.

Forster, A., and Young, J. (1995). Incidence and consequences of falls due to stroke: A systematic inquiry. *BMJ, 311*(6997), 83–86.

Garrett, R., Immink, M. A., and Hillier, S. (2011). Becoming connected: The lived experience of yoga participation after stroke. *Disability and Rehabilitation, 33*(25–26), 2404–2415.

Gerber, G. J., and Gargaro, J. (2015). Participation in a social and recreational day programme increases community integration and reduces family burden of persons with acquired brain injury. *Brain Injury, 29*(6), 722–729.

Grimm, L. A., Van Puymbroeck, M., Miller, K. K., Fisher, T., and Schmid, A. A. (2017). Yoga after traumatic brain injury: Changes in emotional regulation and health-related quality of life in a case-study. *International Journal of Complementary and Alternative Medicine, 8*(1), 00247.

Grossman, G. B. (2015). *Restorative Yoga for Life: A Relaxing Way to De-Stress, Re-Energize, and Find Balance.* Avon, MA: Adams Media.

Hallgren, M., Romberg, K., Bakshi, A. S., and Andréasson, S. (2014). Yoga as an adjunct treatment for alcohol dependence: A pilot study. *Complementary Therapies in Medicine, 22*(3), 441–445.

Hanson, R. (2009). *Buddha's Brain: The Practical Neuroscience of Happiness, Love, and Wisdom.* Oakland, CA: New Harbinger Publications.

Hinsey, K. M., Schmid, A. A., Bolster, R. A., Phillips, C. E., *et al.* (2015). Caregiver burden decreases for caregivers of people with stroke after participating in yoga: A mixed methods study. *International Journal of Yoga Therapy, 25*(S2).

Hölzel, B. K., Carmody, J., Vangel, M., Congleton, C., *et al.* (2011). Mindfulness practice leads to increases in regional brain gray matter density. *Psychiatry Research: Neuroimaging, 191*(1), 36–43.

Immink, M. A., Hillier, S., and Petkov, J. (2014). Randomized controlled trial of yoga for chronic poststroke hemiparesis: Motor function, mental health, and quality of life outcomes. *Topics in Stroke Rehabilitation, 21*(3), 256–271.

Innes, K. E., and Vincent, H. K. (2007). The influence of yoga-based programs on risk profiles in adults with Type 2 Diabetes Mellitus: A systematic review. *Evidence Based Complementary and Alternative Medicine (eCAM), 4*(4), 469–486.

Iyengar, B. (1965). *Light on Yoga.* New York: Schocken Books.

Kerrigan, D. C., Lee, L. W., Collins, J. J., Riley, P. O., and Lipsitz, L. A. (2001). Reduced hip extension during walking: Healthy elderly and fallers versus young adults. *Archives of Physical Medicine and Rehabilitation, 82*(1), 26–30.

Kerrigan, D. C., Todd, M. K., Della Croce, U., Lipsitz, L. A., and Collins, J. J. (1998). Biomechanical gait alterations independent of speed in the healthy elderly: Evidence for specific limiting impairments. *Archives of Physical Medicine and Rehabilitation, 79*(3), 317–322.

Kirkwood, G., Rampes, H., Tuffrey, V., Richardson, J., and Pilkington, K. (2005). Yoga for anxiety: A systematic review of the research evidence. *British Journal of Sports Medicine, 39*(12), 884–891.

Krebs, E., Lorenz, K., Bair, M., Damush, T., *et al.* (2009). Development and initial validation of the PEG, a three-item scale assessing pain intensity and interference. *Journal of General Internal Medicine, 24*(6), 6.

Kristal, A. R., Littman, A. J., Benitez, D., and White, E. (2005). Yoga practice is associated with attenuated weight gain in healthy, middle-aged men and women. *Alternative Therapies in Health and Medicine, 11*(4), 28–33.

Lakkireddy, D., Atkins, D., Pillarisetti, J., Ryschon, K., *et al.* (2013). Effect of yoga on arrhythmia burden, anxiety, depression, and quality of life in paroxysmal atrial fibrillation: The YOGA My Heart Study. *Journal of the American College of Cardiology, 61*(11), 1177–1182.

Lazar, S. W., Bush, G., Gollub, R. L., Fricchione, G. L., Khalsa, G., and Benson, H. (2000). Functional brain mapping of the relaxation response and meditation. *Neuroreport, 11*(7), 1581.

Lazar, S. W., Kerr, C. E., Wasserman, R. H., Gray, J. R., *et al.* (2005). Meditation experience is associated with increased cortical thickness. *Neuroreport, 16*(17), 1893.

Lazaridou, A., Philbrook, P., and Tzika, A. A. (2013). Yoga and mindfulness as therapeutic interventions for stroke rehabilitation: A systematic review. *Evidence-Based Complementary and Alternative Medicine*, doi: 10.1155/2013/357108.

Liepert, J., Miltner, W. H., Bauder, H., Sommer, M., *et al.* (1998). Motor cortex plasticity during constraint-induced movement therapy in stroke patients. *Neuroscience Letters, 250*(1), 5–8.

Lloyd-Billington, M. (2014). Exploring the principles and practices of the yoga tradition. Accessed on 15/04/2018 at www.thelivingyogablog.com.

Lynton, H., Kligler, B., and Shiflett, S. (2007). Yoga in stroke rehabilitation: A systematic review and results of a pilot study. *Topics in Stroke Rehabilitation, 14*(4), 1–8.

Management of Stroke Rehabilitation Working Group. (2010). VA/DOD clinical practice guideline for the management of stroke rehabilitation. *Journal of Rehabilitation Research and Development, 47*(9), 1–43.

Marshall, R. S., Basilakos, A., Williams, T., and Love-Myers, K. (2014). Exploring the benefits of unilateral nostril breathing practice post-stroke: Attention, language, spatial abilities, depression, and anxiety. *The Journal of Alternative and Complementary Medicine, 20*(3), 185–194.

McCall, M. C., Ward, A., Roberts, N. W., and Heneghan, C. (2013). Overview of systematic reviews: Yoga as a therapeutic intervention for adults with acute and chronic health conditions. *Evidence-Based Complementary and Alternative Medicine, 2013*, doi: 10.1155/2013/945895.

McGonigal, K. (2009). *Yoga for Pain Relief: Simple Practices to Calm Your Mind and Heal Your Chronic Pain*. Oakland, CA: New Harbinger Publications.

Miller, K. K., Combs, S. A., Van Puymbroeck, M., Altenburger, P. A., *et al.* (2013). Fatigue and pain: Relationships with physical performance and patient beliefs after stroke. *Topics in Stroke Rehabilitation, 20*, 347–355.

Miller, K. K., Mason, A., Nicolai, N., Altenburger, P., *et al.* (2015). *Gait Speed and Step Parameter Changes After Therapeutic-Yoga in People with Stroke: A Pilot Study*. Paper presented at the American Congress of Rehabilitation Medicine, Dallas, TX.

Mishra, R. S. (1972). *The Textbook of Yoga Psychology: A New Translation and Interpretation of Patanjali's Yoga Sutras for Meaningful Application in All Modern Psychologic Disciplines*. London: Lyrebird Press Ltd.

Moss, A. S., Wintering, N., Roggenkamp, H., *et al.* (2012). Effects of an 8-week meditation program on mood and anxiety in patients with memory loss. *The Journal of Alternative and Complementary Medicine, 18*(1), 48–53.

National Institute on Alcohol Abuse and Alcoholism. (2018). Drinking levels defined. Accessed on 09/05/2018 at www.niaaa.nih.gov/alcohol-health/overview-alcohol-consumption/moderate-binge-drinking.

National Stroke Association (2018) Homepage. Accessed on 09/05/2018 at www.stroke.org.

Newberg, A. B., Wintering, N., Khalsa, D. S., Roggenkamp, H., and Waldman, M. R. (2010). Meditation effects on cognitive function and cerebral blood flow in subjects with memory loss: A preliminary study. *Journal of Alzheimer's Disease, 20*, 517–526.

Okonta, N. R. (2012). Does yoga therapy reduce blood pressure in patients with hypertension? An integrative review. *Holistic Nursing Practice, 26*(3), 137–141.

Page, S. J., and Peters, H. (2014). Mental practice: Applying motor PRACTICE and neuroplasticity principles to increase upper extremity function. *Stroke, 45*(11), 3454–3460.

Page, S. J., Gater, D. R., and Bach-y-Rita, P. (2004). Reconsidering the motor recovery plateau in stroke rehabilitation. *Archives of Physical Medicine and Rehabilitation, 85*(8), 1377–1381.

Page, S. J., Levine, P., and Leonard, A. (2007). Mental practice in chronic stroke results of a randomized, placebo-controlled trial. *Stroke, 38*(4), 1293–1297.

Page, S. J., Schmid, A. A., and Harris, J. (2012). Optimizing language for stroke motor rehabilitation: Recommendations from the ACRM Stroke Movement Interventions Subcommittee. *Archives of Physical Medicine and Rehabilitation, 93*(8), 1395–1399.

Page, S. J., Levine, P., Sisto, S. A., and Johnston, M. V. (2001). Mental practice combined with physical practice for upper-limb motor deficit in subacute stroke. *Physical Therapy, 81*(8), 1455–1462.

Paolucci, S. (2008). Epidemiology and treatment of post-stroke depression. *Neuropsychiatric Disease and Treatment, 4*(1), 145.

Patel, N. K., Newstead, A. H., and Ferrer, R. L. (2012). The effects of yoga on physical functioning and health related quality of life in older adults: A systematic review and meta-analysis. *The Journal of Alternative and Complementary Medicine, 18*(10), 902–917.

Perry, J., Garrett, M., Gronley, J. K., and Mulroy, S. J. (1995). Classification of walking handicap in the stroke population. *Stroke, 26*(6), 982–989.

Pohl, P., Duncan, P., Perera, S., Liu, W., *et al.* (2002). Influence of stroke-related impairments in performance in 6-minute walk test. *Journal of Rehabilitation Research and Development, 39*, 439–444.

Portz, J. D., Waddington, E., Atler, K., Van Puymbroeck, M., and Schmid, A. A. (2016). Self-management and yoga for older adults with chronic stroke: A mixed-methods study of physical fitness and physical activity. *The Clinical Gerontologist, 1*, 1–8.

Prinster, T. (2014). *Yoga for Cancer: A Guide to Managing Side Effects, Boosting Immunity, and Improving Recovery for Cancer Survivors.* New York: Simon and Schuster.

Reddy, S., Dick, A. M., Gerber, M. R., and Mitchell, K. (2014). The effect of a yoga intervention on alcohol and drug abuse risk in veteran and civilian women with posttraumatic stress disorder. *The Journal of Alternative and Complementary Medicine, 20*(10), 750–756.

Rentz, K. (2005). *Yoganap: Relaxation Poses for Deep Relaxation.* Cambridge, MA: Da Capo Press.

Rikli, R., and Jones, C. (2001). *Senior Fitness Test.* Champaign, IL: Human Kinetics.

Rogers, M. W., and Martinez, K. M. (2009). Recovery and Rehabilitation of Standing Balance after Stroke. In J. Stein, R. L. Harvey, R. F. Macko, C. Winstein, and R. D. Zorowitz (Eds.) *Stroke Recovery and Rehabilitation* (evidence table found on p.352). New York: Demosmedical.

Roney, M. A., Sample, P. L., Stallones, L., Van Puymbroeck, M., and Schmid, A. A. (under review). The lived experience of individuals with chronic traumatic brain injury: An adapted group yoga intervention. *International Journal of Yoga Therapy.*

Ruiz, F. P. (2007). Yoga for the eyes. *Yoga Journal*. Accessed on 15/04/2018 at www.yogajournal. com/lifestyle/insight-for-sore-eyes.

Schmid, A. A., and Rittman, M. (2007). Fear of falling: An emerging issue after stroke. *Topics in Stroke Rehabilitation, 14*(5), 46–55.

Schmid, A. A., and Rittman, M. (2009). Consequences of poststroke falls: Activity limitation, increased dependence, and the development of fear of falling. *American Journal of Occupational Therapy, 63*(3), 310–316.

Schmid, A. A., Van Puymbroeck, M., and Koceja, D. M. (2010). Effect of a 12-week yoga intervention on fear of falling and balance in older adults: A pilot study. *Archives of Physical Medicine and Rehabilitation, 91*(4), 576–583.

Schmid, A. A., Acuff, M., Doster, K., Gwaltney-Duiser, A., *et al.* (2009). Poststroke fear of falling in the hospital setting. *Topics in Stroke Rehabilitation, 16*(5), 357–366.

Schmid, A. A., Van Puymbroeck, M., Altenburger, P., Schalk, T., *et al.* (2012). Poststroke balance improves with yoga. *Stroke, 43*(9), 2402–2407.

Schmid, A. A., Van Puymbroeck, M., Altenburger, P. A., Miller, K. K., Combs, S. A., and Page, S. J. (2013a). Balance is associated with quality of life in chronic stroke. *Topics in Stroke Rehabilitation, 20*(4), 340–346.

Schmid, A. A., Yaggi, H., Burrus, N., McClain, V., *et al.* (2013b). Circumstances and consequences of falls among people with chronic stroke. *Journal of Rehabilitation Research and Development, 50*(9), 1277–1286.

Schmid, A. A., Miller, K. K., Van Puymbroeck, M., and DeBaun-Sprague, E. (2014). Yoga leads to multiple physical improvements after stroke: A pilot study. *Complementary Therapies in Medicine, 22*(6), 994–1000.

Schmid, A. A., DeBaun, E., Gilles, A., Maguire, J., Mueller, A., Miller, K. K., and Van Puymbroeck, M. (2014b). *Therapeutic-Yoga Is Complementary to Inpatient Rehabilitation: Patients' Perceived Benefits*. Paper presented at the American Occupational Therapy Association, Baltimore, MD.[AQ]

Schmid, A. A., Arnold, S. E., Jones, V. A., Ritter, M. J., Sapp, S. A., and Van Puymbroeck, M. (2015a). Fear of falling in people with chronic stroke. *The American Journal of Occupation Therapy, 69*(3), 6903350020.

Schmid, A. A., Miller, K. K., Van Puymbroeck, M., and DeBaun-Sprague, E. *et al.* (2015c). Feasibility and results of a pilot study of group occupational therapy for fall risk management after stroke. *British Journal of Occupational Therapy 78*(10), 653–660.

Schmid, A. A., Miller, K. K., Van Puymbroeck, M., and Schalk, N. (2016a). Feasibility and results of a case study of yoga to improve physical functioning in people with chronic traumatic brain injury. *Disability and Rehabilitation, 38*(9), 914–920.

Schmid, A. A., Van Puymbroeck, M., Portz, J. D., Atler, K. E., and Fruhauf, C. A. (2016b). Merging Yoga and Occupational Therapy (MY-OT): A feasibility and pilot study. *Complementary Therapies in Medicine, 28*, 44–49.

Sengupta, P. (2012). Health impacts of yoga and pranayama: A state-of-the-art review. *International Journal of Preventive Medicine, 3*(7), 444.

Shaw, S. (2003). *The Little Book of Yoga Breathing: Pranayama Made Easy…* San Francisco, CA: Weiser Books.

Silverthorne, C., Khalsa, S. B. S., Gueth, R., DeAvilla, N., and Pansini, J. (2012). Respiratory, physical, and psychological benefits of breath-focused yoga for adults with severe traumatic brain injury (TBI): A brief pilot study report. *International Journal of Yoga Therapy, 22*, 47–51.

Stroke Association. (2018). Homepage. Accessed on 09/05/2018 at www.stroke.org.uk.

Stroke Foundation. (2018). Vision loss after stroke fact sheet. Accessed on 09/05/2018 at https:// strokefoundation.org.au/About-Stroke/Help-after-stroke/Stroke-resources-and-fact-sheets/ Vision-loss-after-stroke-fact-sheet.

Truelsen, T., Piechowski-Jóźwiak, B., Bonita, R., Mathers, C., Bogousslavsky, J., and Boysen, G. (2006). Stroke incidence and prevalence in Europe: A review of available data. *European Journal of Neurology, 13*(6), 581–598.

Van Puymbroeck, M., Smith, R., and Schmid, A. A. (2011). Yoga as a means to negotiate physical activity constraints in middle-aged and older adults. *International Journal on Disability and Human Development, 10*(2), 117–121.

Van Puymbroeck, M., Schmid, A., Shinew, K., and Hsieh, P. (2011). Influence of Hatha yoga on the physical fitness, physical activity constraints, and body image of breast cancer survivors: A pilot study. *International Journal of Yoga Therapy, 21*, 81–92.

Van Puymbroeck, M., Allsop, J., Miller, K., and Schmid, A. (2014). ICF-based improvements in body structures and function, and activity and participation in chronic stroke following a yoga-based intervention. *Journal of Recreation Therapy, 13*(3), 23–33.

Van Puymbroeck, M., Miller, K. K., Dickes, L. A., and Schmid, A. A. (2015). Perceptions of yoga therapy embedded in two inpatient rehabilitation hospitals: Agency perspectives. *Evidence-Based Complementary and Alternative Medicine,* doi: 10.1155/2015/125969.

Van Puymbroeck, M., Schmid, A., Walter, A., and Hawkins, B. (2017). Improving leisure constraints in older adults with a fear of falling through Hatha yoga: An acceptability and feasibility study. *International Journal of Gerontology and Geriatric Research, 1*(1), 7–13.

Vennu, V., Kachanathu, S. J., Bhatia, P., and Nuhmani, S. (2013). Efficacy of meditation with conventional physiotherapy management on sub-acute stroke patients. *Scholarly Journal of Medicine, 3*(5), 48–52.

Weerdesteyn, V., de Niet, M., van Duijnhoven, H. J. R., and Geurts, A. C. H. (2008). Falls in individuals with stroke. *Journal of Rehabilitation Research and Development, 45*(8), 1195–1213.

Williams, L., Weinberger, M., Harris, L., and Biller, J. (1999). Measuring quality of life in a way that is meaningful to stroke patients. *Neurology, 53*(8), 1839–1843.

Winstein, C. J., Stein, J., Arena, R., Bates, B., *et al.* (2016). Guidelines for adult stroke rehabilitation and recovery: A guideline for healthcare professionals from the American Heart Association/ American Stroke Association. *Stroke, 47*(6), e98–e169.

Subject Index

Author Index